GUIDELINES FOR OCCUPATIONAL THERAPY PRACTICE IN HOME HEALTH

The American Occupational Therapy Association, Inc.
Bethesda, Maryland 20824-1220

by

The Commission on Practice Home Health Task Force:
Michael J. Steinhauer, OTR, MPH, FAOTA—Chairperson
Rebecca Austill-Clausen, MS, OTR, FAOTA
Judith A. Menosky, MS, OTR/L
Jennifer A. Young, COTA/L
Mary Jane Youngstrom, MS, OTR
Sarah D. Hertfelder, MEd, MOT, OTR—Staff Liaison

with contributions from:

Caroline A. Higgins, OTR/L, CPHQ
Karen Johnson, OTR
Patricia A. Kelly, RN, BSN, OTR
Theodosia T. Kelsey, OTR, FAOTA
Velma Reichenbach, MS, OTR/L

for

The Commission on Practice
Jim Hinojosa, PhD, OTR, FAOTA—Chairperson

For information address: The American Occupational Therapy Association, Inc., 4720 Montgomery Lane, PO Box 31220, Bethesda, MD 20854-1220.

Disclaimers
"This publication is designed to provide accurate and authoritative information in regard to the subject matter covered. It is sold or distributed with the understanding that the publisher is not engaged in rendering legal, accounting, or other professional service. If legal advice or other expert assistance is required, the services of a competent professional person should be sought."
—From the Declaration of Principles jointly adopted by the American Bar Association and a Committee of Publishers and Associations.

It is the objective of the American Occupational Therapy Association to be a forum for free expression and interchange of ideas. The opinions expressed by the contributors to this work are their own and not necessarily those of either the editors or the American Occupational Therapy Association.

Edited by Jennifer A. Irey
Designed by Anthony Rubino, Jr.

Printed in the United States of America

ISBN: 1-56900-023-9

Table of Contents

Preface and Acknowledgments

In 1993, the Commission on Practice (COP) of the American Occupational Therapy Association (AOTA) identified a need to update the 1987 version of *Guidelines for Occupational Therapy Services in Home Health*. This decision was fueled by significant developments in the home health industry: the growth of the industry to new markets including mental health and pediatrics; changing patterns of health care provisions primarily from institutional-based to communicated-based care; the particular role of home health in health care reform proposals; and the consumer demand for home health services. At the same time, AOTA approved the development of the Home and Community Health Special Interest Section. Membership enthusiasm for the Section has been impressive. Further, AOTA's Representative Assembly supported the COP by funding the formation of a Home Health Task Force to update and further enhance this latest publication of *Guidelines for Occupational Therapy in Home Health*.

This document represents the guidelines developed by the Home Health Task Force. They are primarily for those practitioners who work with adult physical disabilities, but guidelines for practice in mental health and pediatric service delivery in the home are also reviewed. The members of the Task Force currently represent a broader scope of practice than the previous committee, including an occupational therapy assistant who is an integral part of the membership. In addition, an academician representing the COP participated in the development of these guidelines.

The guidelines are intended to assist occupational therapists and occupational therapy assistants who are, or are considering, working in home health. As with any method of service delivery, variations exist among home health agencies and programs. The Home Health Task Force has attempted to make the guidelines as comprehensive as possible.

Throughout this document the use of the terms "occupational therapist" and "occupational therapy assistant" have been carefully gauged to reflect appropriate roles and responsibilities for these professions. "Occupational therapy practitioner" is sometimes used to encompass both types. Also, every effort has been extended to ensure compliance with AOTA's *Uniform Terminology for Occupational Therapy—Third Edition*.

The guidelines are rules recommended for practice in home health but they are not binding. Occupational therapy practitioners need to be informed about specific agency policies and procedures; federal, state, and local laws; and professional licensure legislation and regulations. Any of these particular policies, laws, or regulations may negate or revise the general content of these guidelines.

The Home Health Task Force is deeply indebted to the first Home Health Task Force including members Rebecca Austill-Clausen, OTR; Barbara Jackson, OTR; Theodosia T. Kelsey, OTR, FAOTA; Doris Pierce, OTR; and Michael J. Steinhauer, OTR, MPH, for their work related to the publication of the first *Guidelines for Occupational Therapy Services in Home Health*, some of which is the basis for the work in this book. In addition, we are very grateful to Sarah Hertfelder of AOTA's Practice Department, her very able assistant Wendy Schoen, our editor Jennifer Irey, and our current contributing authors and field reviewers. All of them provided valuable assistance without which this document would not have been possible. Finally, the Task Force thank their families who cared for the children and who took on additional responsibilities at home as the members worked on their contributions to this project.

Chapter 1

The Home Health Industry:

Definitions, History, and Types of Service Delivery

by Michael J. Steinhauer,
OTR, MPH, FAOTA

with contributions from
Patricia A. Kelly, RN, BSN, OTR

I. Introduction

The provision of occupational therapy in the home is unique, challenging, rewarding, and exciting. The occupational therapist and the occupational therapy assistant offer a practical and functional service by teaching patients to achieve a maximum level of independence in their familiar surroundings. Occupational therapy practitioners can address the individual's specific functional needs and desires within the context of his or her own unique and personal surroundings. Practitioners in home health also spend a significant amount of their treatment attention on family or caregiver training, and environmental adaptations specific to the patient's needs and surroundings.

As more and more individuals are seen in community settings for health care, the number of occupational therapists and occupational therapy assistants working in home health has steadily increased (American Occupational Therapy Association, 1990). Occupational therapy practitioners make unique contributions to home health by applying their skills in evaluation, function-oriented treatment, and environmental adaptation. With their educational background in psychosocial and physical disabilities, they have the special training needed to treat the patient at home.

A. The Meaning and Culture of Home to the Patient, and the Impact on Collaborative Treatment Planning

The mind-set most useful to a home health practitioner views the patient and their families as the "owners" of the disability experience (Mattingly, 1991). Also taken into consideration is the impact this experience has on their lives. By ascertaining the meaning of home, a practitioner can learn what aspect is important to the patient. Clues to uncover this meaning may be found in the environment, and in their life-styles before illness and during hospitalization. These considerations can help the practitioner design treatment programs to tap into the patient's motivation and their image of themselves after treatment has concluded (Rockwell-Dylla, 1993; Mattingly, 1991).

This theory is particularly true for the melting pot population that characterizes the American landscape of today. Ethnic and cultural differences can greatly influence the relationship of the home health practitioner to the patient and their families. For instance, some families insist on doing all they can to be helpful to the patient without relying on the assistance of professional caregivers. Although the home health frame of reference is to maximize a patient's level of independence so they can do as much for themselves as possible, in these cases the treatment programs may be geared more toward family education than patient independence. As the occupational therapist assesses the patient's strengths and weaknesses in functional performance areas, the practitioner's knowledge, experience, clinical reasoning, and collaborative skills come together to evolve into treatment strategies and outcomes that are "compatible with the client's/caregiver's self-image, belief systems, life-style, and culture" (P.A. Kelly, personal communication, January 1994).

These considerations are especially relevant when the treatment setting is the patient's own residence. It is the uncovering and use of those activities that have meaning and purpose to the patient that will most quickly advance his or her motivation and abilities since "attention, arousal, and motivational inputs are the only way to teach the human brain" (Cool & Oetter, 1990).

As cited in Mattingly (1991), Sir Dominic Corrigan postulated the following regarding physicians: "It's not that they don't know enough, but they don't see enough." In the home health setting, the practitioner might dismiss a client as "therapy not indicated" without eyes and the imagination to see the possibilities of intervention and collaboration. Again, this speaks to the importance of networking with fellow home health practitioners, and for quality supervision to continually expand one's expertise and vision. Both of these methods empower the practitioner to find ways to enhance the lives of even those patients who are at the lowest level of functioning.

Collaborating with interdisciplinary team members and integrating their evaluation information serves to enhance the practitioner's belief in the patient's real possibilities. That belief or vision may catalyze the patient's belief in their own potential, paving the way for activities that can tap into the nervous system's programmability in "selective attention, optimal arousal, and motivational inputs" (Cool & Oetter, 1990). Failure to collaborate with the patient, caregiver, family, and interdisciplinary team to develop interventions and functional outcomes may lead to the patient's resistance, noncompliance, unsuccessful treatment, less than positive view of the health care delivery system, burnout in the practitioner, and a potential for nonreimbursement (P.A. Kelly, personal communication, January 1994).

Even with well-designed intervention strategies and cooperative team collaboration patients,

for reasons of their own, decide what they will do and when and how they will do it (Yerxa, 1991). In home health practice, empowering the patient to keep trying, while revising treatment plans with a focus on working together towards a meaningful goal, is a benchmark to "the extent to which a person respects a plan of action developed through mutual collaboration" (Baker, 1993). Blind compliance by the patient, which suggests a loss of personal ownership, "acquiescence, or a tendency to give into others," is highly discouraged in this sensitive environment where treatment is provided (Guralnick, 1977, p.128). In their own homes, patients have most likely always had a sense of control and ownership in all decisions. Home health practitioners must be sensitive to this therapeutic landscape in order to be successful in providing meaningful treatment interventions.

II. Definitions

A. Clarifying "Home Health" and "Home Care"

The term "home health" or "home care" conjures up many images both to health care professionals and to the layperson. A layperson might think that the latter term means "care of the home" such as periodic household repairs, like the maintenance of gutters and downspouts. Even today, a health care provider might also be at a loss to distinguish between the two terms.

Home health and home care should be considered as two different descriptive terms for services provided at the place of residence of the patient. Traditionally, home health services have a more medically oriented base as the core, whereas home care services are more frequently socially oriented.

Further, the Joint Commission on Accreditation of Healthcare Organizations (1992) defines home health as:

> Services provided by health care professionals in an individual's place of residence on a per-visit or per-hour basis to patients/clients who have or are at risk of an injury, an illness, or a disabling condition or who are terminally ill and require short-term or long-term intervention by health professionals. These services may include dental, medical, nursing, occupational therapy, pediatric, physical therapy, speech-language pathology, audiology, social work, and nutrition counseling services and may be provided directly or through contract with another organization or individual (p.29).

Other definitions of home health provided by health care professional trade organizations, such as the National League of Nurses, closely mimic that of the Joint Commission's.

Home care, however, refers to the support services that complement the health-related services being provided in home health. Examples include homemakers, sitters, companions, telephone reassurance, Meals On Wheels, and friendly visitor services. These support services are not covered by Medicare, but many state public reimbursement sources have programs covering them. Coverage by private insurers varies from policy to policy.

B. Specifying the Term "Homebound" Under Medicare

The documented establishment of a patient's homebound status is critical to assuring eligibility and reimbursement for services. The most commonly employed definition of "homebound" has its roots in Medicare language. The *Medicare Home Health Agency Manual* (Health Care Financing Administration, 1989) defines "homebound" as:

Patient Confined To His Home—In order for a beneficiary to be eligible to receive covered home health services under both Part A and Part B, the law requires that a physician certify in all cases that the beneficiary is confined to his home. An individual does not have to be bedridden to be considered as confined to his home. However, the condition of these patients should be such that there exists a normal inability to leave home and, consequently leaving their homes would require a considerable and taxing effort. If the patient does in fact leave the home, the patient may nevertheless be considered homebound if the absences from the home are infrequent or for periods of relatively short duration, or are attributable to the need to receive medical treatment. Absences attributable to the need to receive medical treatment include attendance at adult day care centers to receive medical care, ongoing receipt of outpatient kidney dialysis, and the receipt of outpatient chemotherapy or radiation therapy. It is expected that in most instances absences from the home that occur will be for the purpose of receiving medical treatment. However, occasional absences from the home for nonmedical purposes (e.g., an occasional trip to the barber, or a walk around the block or a drive) would not necessitate a finding that the individual is not homebound so long as the absences are undertaken on an infrequent basis or are of relatively short duration and do not indicate that the patient has the capacity to obtain the health care provided outside rather than in the home. (Chapter 2, Section 204.1, Subsection A, Transmittal A)

C. Specifying the Term "Intermittent" Under Medicare

It is equally important to understand Medicare's definition of "intermittent" as an eligibility requirement as it is to understand the "homebound" eligibility criteria. Note that the definition of "intermittent" centers around skilled nursing and home health aide services. Occupational therapy practitioners should consider these parameters when designing treatment programs. The *Medicare Home Health Agency Manual* (Health Care Financing Administration, 1989) defines "intermittent" as:

- Up to and including 28 hours per week of skilled nursing and home health aide services combined provided on a less than daily basis;

- Up to 35 hours per week of skilled nursing and home health aide services combined that are provided on a less than daily basis, subject to review by fiscal intermediaries on a case by case basis, based upon documentation justifying the need for and reasonableness of such additional care; or

- Up to and including full-time (i.e., 8 hours per day) skilled nursing and home health aide services combined, which are provided and needed 7 days per week for temporary, but not indefinite, periods of time of up to 21 days with allowances for extensions in exceptional circumstances where the need for care in excess of 21 days is finite and predictable. (Chapter 2, Section 206.7, Subsection B, Transmittal 222)

III. Historical Overview of Home Health

The beginnings of home health in America can be traced back to 1796 at the Boston Dispensary from which laymen provided care to the sick and the poor in their homes. A century later in 1877, the Women's Branch of the New York City Mission hired a graduate nurse to provide home nursing care for the sick. In 1885, the first voluntary nongovernment agency specifically organized to provide nursing care at home was founded in Buffalo, NY. Similar volunteer agencies in Boston and Philadelphia later became known as Visiting Nurse Associations (Stewart, 1979).

As these types of agencies grew, other types of services were added. In 1947, at the Montefiore Hospital in New York, E.M. Bluestone founded a hospital-based home care program called a "hospital without walls" in which treatment was expanded to patients beyond the poor and the elderly (Ryder, 1967). The first mention of occupational therapy in connection with home health occurred in a 1949 article in the *American Journal of Public Health*. Dr. Martin Cherkasky (1949) wrote, "We have a full-time occupational therapist who visits the patient in his home...it is a morale builder and certain corrective procedures can be taught to the patient" (p. 165).

Another landmark in the history of home health was the Conference on Home Care in Roanoke, VA in June 1958. From this conference came a working definition of home care that is the core of policy parameters in home health administration today:

> An organized home care program is a phase of comprehensive medical care given to homebound patients not needing hospitalization, which consists of the following essential elements:
>
> 1. Centralization of responsibility for administration.
>
> 2. A formally structured and coordinated unit comprising at least a physician, a nurse, and a social worker assisted by clerical services that confers periodically with the responsibility to:
>
>> a. carry out admission evaluation of applicants referred to the program;
>>
>> b. plan, review, and modify individual patient service schedules;
>>
>> c. implement and coordinate direct patient services provided by various professions; and
>>
>> d. carry out discharge determinations.
>
> 3. Mobilization of services and resources to provide for individual medical, nursing, social, and rehabilitative needs of each patient within the context of his home and family environment, and supported by necessary inpatient facilities. (American Hospital Association, 1961, pp. 4–5)

A major expansion of home health services came in 1965 after the passage of Title XVIII of the Social Security Act, which is known as Medicare. Trossman (1984) summarized the Act as follows:

> It provides for the aged and disabled. Beneficiaries include people 65 years old and over, people on Social Security Disability for more than 2 years, and individuals needing kidney transplants or dialysis. For a Medicare beneficiary to receive home health care, he or she must (a) be homebound, (b) have services prescribed by and be under the care of a MD, and (c) need part-time or intermittent skilled nursing, physical therapy, or speech therapy. (p. 727)

Until July 1, 1981, home health covered by Medicare was limited to 100 visits in a benefit period, and eligibility under the hospital-insurance component required 3 days of prior hospitalization. The Omnibus Reconciliation Act of 1980, described by Monk (1985), removed these limitations and added occupational therapy as a primary service qualifying for benefits. That law was in effect from July 1, 1981 to December 1, 1981. It was replaced by the Omnibus Budget Reconciliation Act of 1981, which stated:

> Medicare patients may continue to receive occupational therapy services under the home health benefit even after their need for skilled nursing, physical therapy, or speech therapy ends. However, the need for occupational therapy services alone will not qualify them for Medicare home health services. (American Occupational Therapy Association, 1981, p.10)

The same service eligibility criteria exists today.

Occupational therapists may also serve patients in their homes by securing a Medicare provider number and billing for services directly to a fiscal intermediary. A fiscal intermediary, who acts as a liaison, adjudicates the Medicare benefit on behalf of the federal government. Eligible Medicare patients must hold a Part B insurance card and be under the care of a licensed physician.

Medicaid, also known as Title XIX, was created by the Social Security Act of 1965. Medicaid finances health care services to the indigent. It covers hospital and skilled nursing care, home health, physician's services, laboratory work, X rays, and other similar services. Medicaid is different than Medicare in that it does not require "skilled" nursing care or homebound status to be eligible to receive services in the home (Spiegel, 1983).

Additional legislation affecting home health services was the Social Security Amendments of 1983 signed by President Reagan on April 20 of that year. The legislation established a prospective payment system (PPS) based on 468 diagnosis-related groups (DRGs). These apply to the pretreatment diagnosis and related reimbursement categories for all U.S. hospitals reimbursed by Medicare, with the exception of rehabilitation and mental health hospitals. On September 1, 1983, the *Federal Register* published interim final regulations implementing the Medicare DRG's prospective pricing and payment system for hospitals (Caterinicchio, 1984).

The implications of the PPS legislation for the provision of home health have been many, but the primary one is that patients are being discharged "quicker and sicker" ("GAO study", 1985). The hospital now has a monetary incentive to discharge patients sooner, with fewer tests and procedures, than it did before 1983 when all costs were paid for retrospectively.

For the most part, Medicare reimburses home health services and has not undergone substantial changes in its reimbursement parameters since 1983. It can be argued that the only exception occurred in July 1989 when the Health Care Financing Administration (HCFA) issued Transmittal 222 (HCFA, 1989). This transmittal broadened the scope of services already being provided and more clearly delineated, by examples, reimbursement allowances. For instance, Medicare opened an essentially new aspect of reimbursable care by allowing home health practitioners to observe and assess (without direct treatment) a patient's need for possible modification of maintenance programs or an initiation of additional treatment interventions.

As of this writing, it is too early to precisely calculate the structure of the final health care reform initiatives. The legislators are still considering the matter. However, it is clear that the role of home health is likely to be a significant component of any reformed health care system.

IV. Use of Home Health

The National Association for Home Care has compiled a fact sheet on home health that covers expenditures, Medicare involvement, current and projected needs, and sample comparisons of cost for treatment in the home versus other types of care and delivery settings. The fact sheet is updated annually and a recent issuance appears in Appendix A.

V. Types of Service Delivery

Before the enactment of Medicare, most home health was provided by local health departments, Visiting Nurse Associations, and hospital-based programs. Medicare legislation provided a definition of a home health agency (HHA) in the Social Security Act of 1965, which included conditions for this type of agency's participation in Medicare

and Medicaid. HCFA, a division of the Department of Health and Human Services, divided HHAs into five categories in its *Provider Reimbursement Manual* (1986):

1. Combined Official and Voluntary:

   A HHA administered jointly by a voluntary and official agency, supported by tax funds, earnings, and contributions, which provides nursing and therapeutic services.

2. Official (government agency):

   A HHA administered by a state, county, city, or other local unit of government and having as major responsibilities the prevention of disease and community education. The state department of health agencies fall under this category.

3. Voluntary:

   A HHA that is governed by a community-based board of directors and is usually financed by earnings and contributions. The primary function is the care of the sick in their homes. Some voluntary agencies are operated under church auspices. Visiting Nurse Associations often fit into this category.

4. Private Not-for-Profit:

   An HHA that is a privately developed and governed, nonprofit organization other than a Visiting Nurse Association (VNA) that provides care of the sick in the home. This agency must qualify as a tax exempt organization under Title 26 USC 501 (C) of the Internal Revenue Code.

5. Proprietary Organization:

   A HHA owned and operated by an individual or a business corporation. The organization may be a sole proprietorship, partnership (including limited partnership and joint stock company), or corporation. (p. 3201)

Stuart-Siddall (1986) offered this additional description:

Home health agencies are classified further according to location and government structure. Those that are not housed within another type of service delivery system or institution are defined as freestanding; conversely, agencies that are housed within another service delivery system are commonly grouped according to the type of provider. As a result, skilled nursing facility-based (SNF) and hospital-based agencies are common terms within the industry. (p. 24)

Home Health Line (1993), an industry trade news source, provided a summary of home health agencies certified by Medicare as of January 1, 1993. The numbers were compiled by HCFA. The method of categorization has changed over the years:

Visiting Nurse Associations	595
Official	1,193
Rehab-Based	1
Hospital-Based	1,790
Skilled Nursing Facility-Based	107
Proprietary and Non-Profit	2,726 (p. 110)

According to the above numbers, "while the number of Medicare certified agencies fell nearly 5 percent, the number of hospital-based agencies was up 17 percent in the period 1986-1989. Hospital-based HHA's now account for 28 percent of all Medicare-certified agencies, up from 21 percent in 1986" (HCFA, 1993, p.110).

Besides these agencies, many prepaid systems providing health services, such as health maintenance organizations (HMOs) and preferred provider organizations (PPOs), have developed their own home health programs or have contracted with home health agencies to provide care. In addition, home health is provided through state departments of public welfare (e.g., community mental health/mental retardation centers).

VI. Conclusion

Today the home health industry is strong, growing, and acknowledged as a viable complement to the acute care needs addressed traditionally by institutional care facilities. Today, and especially in the near future as health care reform looms, home health practice will enjoy a significant role in health care provisions through managed care systems. With consumer demand for home health and home health practice evolving over the years to adapt to the demands of the communities we serve, the profession of occupational therapy could not find a better "home."

Occupational therapists and occupational therapy assistants have a wide range of opportunities awaiting them in the home health practice arena. There are many employment settings where occupational therapy practitioners can exercise their professional skills and have a dramatic impact on the health and well-being of their patients.

References

American Hospital Association. (1961). *Home care* (Hospital Monograph Series No. 9). Chicago: Author.

American Occupational Therapy Association. (1990). *1990 member data survey summary report*. Rockville, MD: Author.

American Occupational Therapy Association. (1981, September). The Omnibus Budget Reconciliation Act of 1981. *Federal Report* (special edition), No. 81–1. Rockville, MD: Author.

Baker, D. B. (1993). *Predicting and preventing falls in the elderly*. Speech given at the National Home Care Nursing Conference. Conference sponsored by Contemporary Forum, Chicago, IL.

Caterinicchio, R. (1984). *DRGs: What they are and how to survive them*. Thorofare, NJ: Slack.

Cherkasky, M. (1949). The Montefiore Hospital home care program. *American Journal of Public Health, 39,* 163–169.

Cool, S., and Oetter, P. (1990). *Preconference institute on neurobiology and development*. Conducted at the American Occupational Therapy Association Annual Conference, New Orleans, LA.

GAO study on Medicare's new prospective payment system flags potential hazards for older Americans. (1985, Spring). *Aging Reports*, p.2.

Guralink, D. B. (Ed.). (1977). *Webster's new American dictionary*. New York: Popular Library.

HCFA claims 48 new "official" HHAs and 45 new Visiting Nurse Associations. (1993, March). *Home Health Line*, p. 110.

Health Care Financing Administration. (1989). *Medicare home health agency manual*. Washington, DC: Department of Health and Human Services.

Health Care Financing Administration. (1986). *Provider reimbursement manual*. Chicago: Commerce Clearing House.

Joint Commission on Accreditation of Healthcare Organizations. (1992). *Accreditation manual for home care* (Vol. 1 Standards). Oakbrook Terrace, IL: Author.

Mattingly, C. (1991). The narrative nature of clinical reasoning. *American Journal of Occupational Therapy, 45* (11), 998–1005.

Monk, A. (1985). *A handbook of gerontological services*. New York: Van Nostrand Reinhold.

Rockwell-Dylla, L. (1993, October). *Older adult's meaning of environment: Hospital and home*. Paper presented at the Illinois Occupational Therapy Association Conference, Hillside, IL.

Ryder, C.F. (1967). *Changing patterns in home care* (PHS Publication No. 1657). Washington, DC: Public Health Service.

Spiegel, A.D. (1983). *Home health care*. Owings Mills, MD: National Health Publishing.

Stewart, J.E. (1979). *Home health care*. St. Louis: C.V. Mosby.

Stuart-Sidall, S. (1986). *Home health care nursing*. Gaithersburg, MD: Aspen Systems.

Trossman, P.B. (l984). Administrative and professional issues for the occupational therapist in home health care. *American Journal of Occupational Therapy, 38,* 726–733.

Yerxa, E. J. (1991). Nationally speaking: Seeking a relevant, ethical, and realistic way of knowing for occupational therapy. *American Journal of Occupational Therapy, 45* (2), 201.

Chapter 2

Home Health Practice

Considerations for the Practitioner

by Michael J. Steinhauer,
OTR, MPH, FAOTA

I. Introduction

This chapter is divided into three sections beginning with the community-based treatment setting of home health and the different professional expectations and personal demands made on practitioners. The most compatible personal characteristics of individuals who are considering working in home health are explored so that practitioners can match their own characteristics with those suggested. In this way, a practitioner can determine the likelihood of success and satisfaction in the home health setting.

Second, competency issues are addressed. How can practitioners best prepare themselves for home health practice? How do home health practitioners identify weaknesses in their clinical knowledge base, and how do they seek ongoing supervision? Further, what experience is necessary to assure that one's clinical skills will be sufficient to meet the demands of this setting?

Third, ethics and professional behavior are discussed in broad terms focusing on home health practitioners and issues unique to the relative isolation they face when an ethical issue or a challenge to their professional behavior arises. Current agency and industry trends will also be discussed in this section.

II. Personal Skills and Characteristics

Unique demands in home health dictate certain personality characteristics for occupational therapists and occupational therapy assistants to consider in determining their ability to function effectively in this area of practice. Independence, flexibility, adaptability, and ingenuity are all necessary personal ingredients for home health field personnel. There is limited on-site supervision or peer contact in home health relative to institutional settings, so emergencies, conflicts between patients and their families, and tensions with other staff members must be handled independently. Further, flexibility is required to deal with weather, unpleasant home conditions, transportation difficulties, and scheduling problems.

Many tasks involved in home health, aside from patient care, are very time- consuming. Note writing is a prime example. It can be easily accomplished by using one of several techniques including becoming familiar with personal computers, a dictaphone machine, or use of a personal secretary or typing service. Note that the use of a service or a secretary requires arrangements for dropping off, picking up, duplicating, and signing notes in order for the system to be effective and assure good time management.

Note writing in front of the patient, other than jotting down information to be enhanced later, has the potential to cause concern and resentment on the parts of both the homebound patient and the caregivers who both may feel that this is time that could have otherwise been spent on treatment of the patient. In addition, writing notes in front of the patient may not be advised because it may reinforce the concepts of professional authority rather than the interactive rapport characteristic that is important for practitioners in any setting, particularly in the patient's home. Many occupational therapists and occupational therapy assistants write notes outside their patient's home immediately following a visit in order to reduce the documentation demand on their patient's time.

On the other hand, there are agencies that encourage note writing in the patient's home so that a more precise document can be prepared while fresh in the practitioner's mind. The patient also has the opportunity to cosign the note. The cosigning idea not only verifies the actual treatment provided but also allows for the patient's full participation in treatment. Clearly, home health agencies employ differing policies or practices that should be reviewed to assure compliance.

Another time-consuming skill required by home health practitioners is treatment planning. Home health treatment planning requires telephoning the physician and team members, investigating community resources by telephone or visitation, and locating and purchasing equipment or adaptations to facilitate the patient's independence. These important aspects of quality care can disrupt schedules, and the home health practitioner must incorporate these inconveniences with a calm and highly organized planning attitude.

Scheduling and coordinating visits with other professionals, aides, and family members around their regular routines may further complicate matters. Consecutive treatment services can be fatiguing for both the patient and family.

In home health it is important for the occupational therapy practitioner to consider the focus of each visit. If bathing and dressing are the areas being addressed, a visit at the time the patient prefers or is used to bathing is more appropriate than scheduling bath training for 4:00 p.m. Another consideration in scheduling is knowing when a caregiver will be available to be trained to carry out the occupational therapy program or when the home health aide will be in the home to be instructed.

It is important to remember that the schedules of home health practitioners are not limited solely to patient contact. A typical treatment schedule is based on an 1 hour per patient treatment ratio that does not include travel time. Usually an average direct-treatment sessions lasts 45–50 minutes, leaving 10–15 minutes for note writing.

Other important characteristics that are essential for a considerate and valued practitioner are reliability and regularity. These traits help to build an atmosphere of trust and confidence in the home health program. In this regard, scheduling patients to allow maximum hours for treatment and minimum hours for driving is imperative for effective time management. One must be flexible to plan for a patient's appointments with his or her physician, new referrals, and associated evaluations, which often come up without notice, while maintaining a continuous flow of treatment hours throughout the day. When possible, it is suggested that occupational therapists and occupational therapy assistants stay within a 25 mile radius of their agency or home, or try to limit territories to a maximum of 30–40 minutes driving time between patients in order to maximize their time. Ideally when applying for a position with a home health agency, the matter of assigned territories should be discussed.

III. Safety

Another consideration for the home health practitioner is safety. Most agencies have some procedure for maintaining contact with practitioners in the field for scheduling and safety purposes. It is a good idea to have contact with other agency field personnel such as the nurse or physical therapist to gain insight on safety considerations for a particular area. Some agencies provide an escort service in high risk areas. Neighborhood watch groups and the crime prevention staff of local police departments are good resources for assistance. Local police departments can also give specific information about their catchment area. The following are some tips that may be helpful to occupational therapy practitioners in the field (Bittel, 1986):

- Carry two sets of car keys.

- Dress in complete uniform if required by the agency.

- Wear only minimal jewelry. If possible, avoid carrying a purse, but if necessary keep the purse under the car seat or locked in the trunk while driving.

- During the home visit, use a small wallet/purse and carry it hidden in a pocket.

- Carry a limited amount of money in a money clip. If accosted, throw it away and run in the opposite direction, yelling in a loud voice if necessary.

- Don't remain in the field after the assigned time.

- Check in with the office regularly and if possible, have the patients who are scheduled for the day call the office if you are very late in meeting at the scheduled appointment time.

- Visit patients only at the addresses assigned and in the order scheduled.

- Don't enter a building that appears unsafe. Carefully look around to discourage any potential assailant time alone with you.

- Establish a travel plan for the area to be visited before leaving the office.

- Use caution when entering an elevator or hallway. In an elevator, stay near the buttons and press every one if necessary. Get off the elevator if you are worried.

- Look in and around your car before entering; keep valuables out of sight.

- Stay alert and act confident.

- Visit high-risk areas as early in the day as possible.

In addition, it is advised that automobiles be well-maintained and that practitioners in this practice setting join auto assistance programs or motor clubs for service in the event of car breakdown. If expenses allow, the use of a cellular phone for emergencies may provide some comfort for personal security. Name tags are also highly suggested in the field.

IV. Achieving Competency

In these days of rapid changes in the health care system, occupational therapy practitioners may feel attracted to the higher salaries and flexible hours associated with home health, which is one of the most rapidly expanding industries in the United States (Halamandaris, 1991). Home health, however, offers significant challenges and a different mindset from the type of practice found successful in hospital and clinic settings (Rockwell-Dylla, 1993). Home health demands a greater

reliance on one's own ethical core, dedication to the expansion of clinical reasoning skills, and the humility to take all the necessary steps to ask for help, seek supervision, and secure second opinions to validate treatment plans and implementation strategies. These efforts enhance the exchange of information and experiences that can provide the validation and support needed to maintain a high level of ability to provide competent care as well as assuring one's own wellness and enthusiasm for the work being performed.

As with all occupational therapy practice in any setting, practitioners should not accept referrals if it is deemed that the patient presents problems that are unfamiliar and that may take some time to ensure appropriate consultation with more experienced colleagues.

Practitioners should be sure that their abilities to assess and treat a wide range of diagnostic groups is adequate, and that they can treat the type of patient most common to the agency where they work. Also, the competent practitioner in home health will establish an effective method for securing adaptive and durable medical equipment from local vendors.

A. Continuing Education

The home health arena is an area of practice for experienced practitioners because of the complexity of issues involved such as acuity of illness, multidiagnoses, multiethnicity, variable family dynamics, codependency, service to primarily a geriatric population, the potential of interdisciplinary team conflicts, and the relative isolation of the home health practitioner. Competence should be founded on a broad knowledge and experience basis, coupled with an acceptance of human behavior and nature as manifested in the patient's own environment.

Retooling professional skills with continuing education to upgrade knowledge and skills is an integral part of the responsibility of being a home health professional. Practitioners are bound by a professional sense of duty and a code of ethics to keep informed on how to deliver the highest quality care possible. Ongoing continuing education may be the financial responsibility of the occupational therapy practitioner and should not be neglected. Practitioners should expect to continue to regularly refurbish their expertise, regardless of background and experience. Therapists who come to home health with a specialty background such as pediatrics or mental health, may need further education to prepare for competence in physical disabilities or in geriatrics. In addition, for those practitioners in private practice, a basic knowledge of business methods is advised, including the issue of varying tax consequences in setting up a practice. It is essential to try and seek out a supportive home health agency environment where continuing education is encouraged, and sensitivity to placing patients in the care of competent staff is important.

The home health industry is continually challenged by the urgent need for competent occupational therapy practitioners. Specific standards for competency have yet to be developed by the home health industry. As practitioners continue to enter the field, opportunities will exist to help shape the selection process.

B. Achieving Competency: Additional Methods

The home health practitioner represents their profession to the local community, home health agency, medical community, interdisciplinary team, and patients. A professional appearance, knowledge base, dependability, timeliness, communication skills, and enthusiasm all reflect on the individual practitioner and the profession as a whole. As stated earlier, home health practitioners generally manage their own schedules, referrals, treatment plans and interventions, documentation, clinical techniques, and professional relations with limited support from departmental peers.

To ensure the greatest level of competency possible, practitioners should consider these suggestions:

- Participate fully in all orientation and in-service programs offered by the agency, covering material that includes, but is not limited to, clinical and administrative policies, universal precautions and infection control, quality assurance/improvement of personnel policies, reimbursement parameters, documentation requirements, supervision availability, emergency preparedness and procedures, incident reporting, appropriate forms use, frequency of scheduled meetings, patient rights and responsibilities, and safety programs.
- Network with the local, state, and national occupational therapy associations for continuing education workshops, self-study courses, and competency self-assessment tools as developed by the American Occupational Therapy Association (AOTA).
- Participate in the local home health special interest sections of occupational therapy associations.
- Develop a library of resource materials to assist in assuring that all aspects of care are being considered when developing treatment plans.
- Be acutely aware of community resources to aid the patient after discharge from the home health program. Discuss good resources with the social worker.

Professional competency in home health generally rests with the individual therapist, the commitment to patients, the organizations served, and themselves. A competent occupational therapist can establish credibility and provide meaning and effectiveness in the provision of services.

C. Experience Needed

New Graduates: New graduates are discouraged from entering the field of occupational therapy in home health. The home health practice environment contains too many demands that can generally only be satisfied by experienced practitioners. However, home health agencies and staffing organizations pursue new graduates with great vigor due to shortages of occupational therapy practitioners around the country. If the new graduate has had previous exposure to home health practice via affiliations or volunteer work, and the level of supervision offered by the home health agency is consistent, on-site as necessary, and provided by an occupational therapist, it is possible to achieve the appropriate amount of experience necessary for a successful tenure in home health.

New graduate-certified occupational therapy assistants may generally be guided by the same criteria as occupational therapists when considering employment in home health.

Experienced Practitioners: Occupational therapy practitioners who have been practicing in other settings may be best advised to consider themselves as entry-level when considering home health as a new field. They should consult and comply with the recommendations cited in the AOTA's publication entitled *Occupational Therapy Roles* (1993). This document clearly outlines role descriptions, supervision issues, qualifications of both occupational therapists and occupational therapy assistants, and key performance areas that specify common activities and expectations associated with role function. In addition, the Home Health Task Force recommends a minimum of 1 year of experience in a physical disability setting with exposure to a wide variety of diagnostic groups.

Since the occupational therapist is ethically responsible and legally accountable for the treatment given by the certified occupational therapy assistant being supervised, the occupational therapist must also establish the assistant's competency levels before allowing them a caseload of their own. Occupational therapy assistants are advised to consult and abide by *Occupational Therapy Roles* (AOTA, 1993) with the knowledge that the Home Health Task Force recommends no less than 2 years experience in a physical disability setting with exposure to a wide variety of diagnostic groups.

V. Ethics and Professional Behavior

The study of bioethics and ethics in health care is currently recognized by policymakers, practitioners, and in the consumer community. For example, the 1993 standards manual issued by the Joint Commission on Accreditation of Healthcare Organizations (JCAHO, 1993), required agencies to formally address ethical issues in home health for the first time. Although these standards are to be updated in the 1995 edition of the *Accreditation Manual for Home Care*, addressing ethical issues will still be required.

A. Occupational Therapy Code of Ethics—American Occupational Therapy Association

AOTA published *Occupational Therapy Code of Ethics* (1994), which should be standard reading material for all practitioners. A copy should be kept available for reference with other important documents. The principles of the document include beneficence/autonomy, competence, compliance with laws and regulations, public information (accurately representing occupational therapy services), and professional relationships and conduct. In addition, the Code references enforcement procedures that have been developed for the investigation and adjudication of alleged violations. The enforcement procedures protect both the profession as well as individual practitioners by setting standard guidelines for practice and ethical and legal issues.

In home health, addressing ethical issues and assuring appropriate professional behavior takes on a special demand. Since the practice of home health is relatively isolated, a practitioner in this practice setting may often not have a support system of fellow practitioners to consult. As a result,

when there is a dilemma, practitioners are generally guided only by his or her own sense of right and wrong. However, in the arena of ethical considerations, right and wrong can take on meanings greater than that of just morality and one's own value system. For example, the complex area of health law including federal, state, and local regulations can all have an influence on decisions. Issues may include matters related to advance directives, standards of practice, public representation issues, uncertainties about professional relationships, and a host of other considerations.

B. Home Health Agency's Ethics Committee

Many home health agencies have established ethics committees to help resolve issues brought to attention by the staff, or to assist patients and their families with difficult health care decisions. However, before formal case consultations with patients and families can be offered, an ethics committee must be properly educated and prepared. The purchase of books, subscriptions to journals that focus on bioethics, memberships in health care ethics societies, and attendance at national and local conferences are necessary expenditures to ensure a well-informed committee.

Educating home health agency staff members is also a critical aspect of the process. They must know how to gain access to the committee, when consultation with the committee is appropriate, and when resolving issues should only be between the practitioner and his or her supervisor.

Community members such as patient advocates, members of the clergy, and consumers should actively participate in the ethics committee. Occupational therapists and occupational therapy assistants should participate as well.

Ethics committees should reach out to families and caregivers of current patients on the agency's roster to encourage their participation in addressing ethical issues that may have arisen during the patient's care. Some of the issues raised at an ethics committee may involve:
- Confidentiality and privacy.
- Determining capacity and competence for decision making.
- Informed consent for treatment.
- Informed refusal for treatment.
- Foregoing life-sustaining treatment.
- Issues related to access to health care.
- Costs and allocation of limited resources.
- Issues related to professional or agency misconduct.

- Exploring conflicting values that arise in individual cases or in agency policies.

The mere presence of an ethics committee serves to encourage a positive, conscious effort to resolve problems and prevent them from occurring in the future. Tools such as a Code of Ethics and ethics committees improve the quality of decisions made by staff and administration.

Each therapist must assume responsibility for the Code of Ethics by which business and professional care is conducted. Supporting ethical practices and seeking consultation for difficult decisions helps chart a course of self-evaluation and rewards the patients, agencies, and the practitioners themselves with an integrity-based culture of uncompromised quality service.

References

American Occupational Therapy Association. (1994). *Occupational therapy code of ethics.* Rockville, MD: Author.

American Occupational Therapy Association. (1994). *Reference manual of official documents.* Rockville, MD: Author.

American Occupational Therapy Association. (1993). *Occupational therapy roles.* Rockville, MD: Author.

Bittel, E.M. (1986). Safety tips for the community health nurse in urban practice. *Home Health Care Nurse, 4,* 30–3l.

Halamandaris, V. (1991). The power of caring. *Caring Magazine, 10* (10), pp. 4–10.

Joint Commission on Accreditation of Healthcare Organizations. (1992). *Accreditation manual for home care—1993* (Volume 1, Standards). Oakbrook Terrace, IL: Author.

Rockwell-Dylla, L. (1993). *Older adult's meaning of environment: Hospital and home.* Paper presented at the Illinois Occupational Therapy Association Conference, Hillside, IL.

Chapter 3

Teamwork, Personnel Issues, and Supervision in the Home Health Setting

by Jennifer A. Young, COTA/L, and
Mary Jane Youngstrom, MS, OTR

I. Introduction

Teamwork is very important to home health. It forms the background against which decisions are made about patient care. Through active team effort, positive patient outcomes can be maximized. Because of the nature of the service delivery process in home health, teamwork does not always occur easily and naturally. Willingness to reach out to each other and facilitate interaction are important responsibilities of each team member.

II. Importance of Communication and Collaboration

The nature of home health service delivery requires that team members treat patients alone at various times of the day throughout the week. This system maximizes the patient's treatment time with care providers and allows for periodic, yet regular, contact. However, this disjointed approach can make communication among team members and monitoring of patient status problematic. Each team member needs to be aware of the multiple areas that other members are treating. Monitoring the patient's response and communicating this information to the appropriate team member is an important responsibility. For example, the occupational therapy practitioner should be sensitive to the patient's response to medications and communicate with the nurse and physician as appropriate. Not being aware of the care the patient may be receiving from others can hinder progress and deprive the patient of a coordinated, therapeutic approach.

Generally, each discipline independently schedules their service with the exception of joint or supervisory visits. Infrequent personal contact among team members necessitates that other methods of communication be established such as by phone, pager, or voice mail. These tools help with scheduling, resolving of scheduling conflicts, and decreasing the likelihood of two disciplines arriving to treat the patient at the same time, which may or may not be reimbursable.

Joint visits involving two disciplines such as occupational therapy and physical therapy or between the registered occupational therapist (OTR) and the home health aide may occasionally occur. Such visits are helpful for coordination and communication and can enhance the patient's overall treatment program. However, when two disciplines see the patient during the same time period it is important that each discipline provide direct service to the patient that is distinct from the service provided by the cotreating discipline. This difference must be reflected in the documentation. A clear delineation of the service of each discipline will help to insure proper reimbursement. Different agencies may also have specific policies regarding joint visits. It is important to check with the individual agency regarding regulations.

Written communication between team members can occur by reading progress notes from other disciplines and visit logs kept in the patient's home. It may be helpful to highlight significant changes or information in the notes to draw attention to anything that could impact treatment provided by other disciplines. Scheduling overlapping visits may sometimes also be arranged. The practitioner should be knowledgeable of when other home health practitioners are visiting and aware of how occupational therapy treatment integrates with the other disciplines' treatment programs.

Some agencies hold staff meetings that vary in frequency from once a week to bimonthly. At these meetings, new patients, problem patients, and general policies may be discussed. Occupational therapy practitioners who are employees of the home health agency are generally required to attend. Independent contractors may or may not be required to attend, and may or may not be paid for attending depending on how their contracts are written. Individuals who are independent contractors should realize that attending staff meetings may be extremely beneficial in enhancing teamwork and should consider attending, even if it is not a requirement.

Not to be overlooked in the home health setting is the importance of regular communication and collaboration with the family and caregivers. Treatment that occurs in the home takes place in the family's "territory." Although the practitioner enters the setting with the authority of knowledge and expertise, the family and patient are still "in charge." In their own homes, patients and families have a stronger sense of control and ownership of all decisions. Collaborating with the family and patient to develop meaningful goals and activities is the primary method for ensuring follow-through, cooperation, and successful outcomes.

Agencies may differ in the types and frequency of team communication that is required of home health practitioners. Whatever the requirements, the practitioner must always keep in mind the importance of communicating the patient's status to the case manager and other appropriate team members. Because patients are seen alone and at different times by the various disciplines, other team members need to be apprised of changes which may occur in between their visits.

III. Types of Team Models— Multidisciplinary and Interdisciplinary

Teams can be organized in different ways. The two most common structures in the home health setting are the multidisciplinary and interdisciplinary models. In both models, the patient is evaluated individually and treatment is implemented by each discipline. However, the approaches differ in terms of the method and type of communication that occurs during the program planning and service delivery process.

In the multidisciplinary model, the various disciplines may share information but no formal attempt is made to coordinate resources or efforts. Disciplines are aware of each other's work but continue their own efforts in relative isolation. In the interdisciplinary model, more formal communication occurs. Generally, a case manager is assigned to a patient's case to coordinate care and avoid fragmentation of services. Team meetings occur where disciplines share information and develop "team" treatment goals and plans. Individual disciplines may find that their own goals and plans become somewhat modified by the team's input. However, as in the multidisciplinary model, treatment implementation still occurs individually and in an isolated manner.

In reality, teams may function anywhere along the continuum between these two approaches. The practical constraints of workload and schedules may complicate the development of a pure interdisciplinary model, but elements of the model may be combined with those of the multidisciplinary approach.

IV. Case Management

Case management in the home health setting involves the coordination and monitoring of the various services that the patient is receiving. Because services are provided individually and care providers may have limited or irregular opportunities to see each other, it is important to have one individual who funnels critical information and service needs. Although one individual may be designated as the case manager, each team member still retains responsibility for care coordination of their own service with that of the other disciplines. The case manager provides the individual service providers with an additional and overall resource for case coordination.

The case manager serves as the liaison between the patient, family, and service providers. He or she will open and close the case, coordinate ongoing services, and advocate for needed services. In the home health setting, the case manager is usually the nurse, however other professionals may also serve in this role. The case manager should be contacted regularly with pertinent information on changes in the patient's condition, progress, and type and frequency of service. Overall changes in the patient's rehabilitation potential also need to be reported and discussed with the case manager.

V. Definitions/Role Descriptions

The team in the home health setting comprises the same members who work in the traditional hospital setting. The following brief descriptions will clarify the roles of the various team members in the home health setting and describe how the occupational therapy practitioner works with each team member.

A. Certified Occupational Therapy Assistant (COTA)

The occupational therapy assistant (COTA), under the supervision of the occupational therapist, can be an effective therapeutic agent in home health. After an OTR has conducted an evaluation and established the treatment plan and goals, the COTA's unique role is to carry out the treatment program. The COTA may treat patients on-site without the physical presence of the occupational therapist. The COTA provides treatment activities to improve abilities in identified performance areas and components with the final goal of returning the patient to the optimal level of independent functioning within the home. When service competency has been established by the OTR and the COTA, the COTA may also administer standard-ized tests in a noninterpretive manner with the OTR's supervision. Other aspects of the COTA's role include assisting in activities of daily living (ADL) evaluation, ordering of equipment, providing adaptations to equipment and the environment, and training caregivers.

B. Family

Today, more than ever, it is essential that the family as well as the patient be closely involved from the beginning in the rehabilitation treatment process. With overstressed family systems often being the norm, lack of family input or involvement in goal setting can negatively influence patient and family commitment to the treatment program. The family and caregivers are crucial team members in providing reinforcement and support for the patient and in encouraging progress.

In assessing who will be available to care for the patient and follow through with the therapy program, the home health practitioner should consider the mental and physical capabilities of the designated caregiver. For example, if the person has a cardiac problem, has had recent surgery, or suffers from an acute condition such as a rheumatoid arthritis flare-up, his or her physical ability to carry out the occupational therapy program may be affected. In addition, the caregiver's cognitive abilities also need to be evaluated so that the practitioner can determine the type and degree of involvement that will be possible and safe.

C. Home Health Aide

The use of home health aides has expanded in the home health practice setting as families have become less available and open to participation. Medicare requires that home health aides be formally trained. Part of the aide's training program includes an orientation to occupational therapy and an understanding of how the aide may work with the occupational therapy practitioner.

The home health aide assists the patient with a variety of personal care tasks such as bathing, grooming, and dressing. The aide monitors the patient's condition by checking the skin and vital signs, and looking for medication side effects. Home health aides should not be confused with homemakers, chore helpers, sitters, or companions whose roles are to provide support services such as doing laundry, preparing meals, or reading to the patient. These types of services are not reimbursed under Medicare but may be funded by other plans, community agencies, or private funds.

D. Licensed Practical Nurse (LPN)

A licensed practical nurse (LPN) will usually see the patient in between the registered nurse's (RN) visits. The LPN monitors patients just like the RN and treats patients in accordance with the nursing practice act in their state. However, he or she must be supervised by the RN. Not all agencies use LPNs and variations in their duties may exist among agencies.

E. Mental Health Registered Nurse

Some agencies also employ nurses on staff who have specialized training or previous experience in mental health nursing. The mental health RN can be helpful in treating a variety of patients since any illness can affect the mental health well-being. The qualification of the mental health RN requires approval by the fiscal intermediary in order to be reimbursed by Medicare.

F. Occupational Therapist (OTR)

The OTR focuses on the patient's overall ability to function in the home and to resume the activities and roles that are important to the individual. The OTR's role includes an initial evaluation of the patient's abilities and the development of the treatment plan and goals. The evaluation identifies performance problems in ADL, work, productive activities (including home management and care of others), and leisure activities. Also identified are specific performance deficits that impact performance areas including sensory, perceptual, cognitive, neuro-musculoskeletal, motor, or psychosocial. Evaluation in the home setting allows the therapist to observe the actual context in which performance will occur and to translate improvement in performance deficits into meaningful everyday tasks. Safety issues, family training, and environmental modifications can also be easily addressed. Either the OTR or COTA, under the supervision of an OTR, may carry out the treatment program. However, according to Medicare, the OTR must conduct the discharge visit.

Safety issues in performance and environmental modifications needed to support performance are readily evident when treating in the home and can be addressed directly. Because of the presence of and easy access to the caregiver, home health treatment often includes teaching the family appropriate support techniques and strategies that will assist in the patient's independence.

G. Physical Therapist (PT)

Physical therapists (PT) and occupational therapy practitioners may work very closely together in the treatment of home health patients. The PT generally focuses on ambulation/mobility, dynamic/static balance, extremity strength, range of motion, and overall endurance. Gains made in physical therapy can often be incorporated into meaningful activities by the OTR that enhance the patient's ability to perform in the home setting. It is often advantageous and advisable to schedule an overlapping visit with the PT to confer and observe treatment given by each discipline. This method enables each discipline to integrate similarities into their program for reinforcement and sharper focus on problem resolution. Coordination of the efforts of these two disciplines is important to assure quality care, avoid duplication, and provide the best treatment outcome.

H. Physician

On occasion a physician may make a home visit, but this is not the norm. The physician's role on the home health team is to initially refer and approve the plan of care and then to reevaluate the plan at least every 60 days in accordance with Medicare regulations or as often as required by a third-party payer. Significant changes in the patient's medical condition or questions should be directed to the physician. Updates should be sent to the physician as often as indicated or required by third-party payers or regulators.

I. Registered Nurse (RN)

In the home, the RN carries out nursing functions similar to those provided in other settings including the monitoring of basic medical status (e.g. blood pressure, blood sugar), and medication compliance and reactions. The RN gives insulin shots, provides wound care, and changes catheters. As previously discussed, the RN may also function as the case manager.

J. Social Worker

The social worker serves in a supportive role to the patient and family. The occupational therapy practitioner should be aware of the social worker as a resource person for the family and also as an individual who can assist in locating needed community information. Social workers can obtain financial resources, locate community transportation, and assist in making referrals to other community agencies such as day care centers. The occupational therapy practitioner can provide useful information to the social worker in reference to the patient's ability to utilize community resources.

K. Speech-Language Pathologist

The speech-language pathologist works with the patient to develop needed speech and language skills and the cognitive processes to support communication. The speech-language pathologist and occupational therapy practitioner share concern for the patient's performance in the areas of cognition, visual perception, and oral motor functioning (i.e., feeding). When both disciplines are treating the same deficit area, documentation needs to delineate the difference in treatment goals. A coordinated approach can often benefit the patient and improve overall performance.

L. Miscellaneous Services

Podiatrists, dentists, prosthetists, and even beauticians do visit patients in the home environment. When working with the developmentally delayed population in the home setting, the teacher may also be an important team member. Developing a list of professionals who will provide needed services in the home is a helpful resource for the home health practitioner. Being able to connect the patient with needed services can facilitate recovery and encourage reestablishment of normal community involvement.

VI. The Occupational Therapy Team

Although OTRs often work in the home health setting without the assistance of COTAs, the development of an OTR/COTA team can expand the availability of service to patients. As in any other setting, service competency must be established between the OTR and the COTA (AOTA, 1987). Ongoing and regular communication is vital to efficient and effective care.

The roles of the OTR and the COTA are the same in this setting as in other settings. Typically in the home care environment, the OTR conducts the initial evaluation and establishes the treatment goals and plan. After the OTR's initial visit, the OTR and COTA hold a case conference that is documented (see Chapter 8 on documentation). After the case conference, the COTA begins to carry out the treatment program. The COTA, on subsequent visits, may collect data to update goals and care plans and may add to assessment data in certain areas. Criterion referenced tests, such as ADL evaluations, may also be conducted after the establishment of service competency. The OTR and COTA collaborate to formulate the discharge plan. The

OTR, however, must complete the discharge visit, according to the Medicare guidelines.

VII. Supervision

In home health, all levels of practitioners should recognize that ongoing supervision is a necessary component of the practice setting. Supervision is sought to maintain individual competence, keep abreast of current trends in practice, solve problems, and develop professional networking. The supervision needs and relationships of the home health aide, COTA, and OTR are discussed in the following section of this chapter.

A. Home Health Aides

Supervision and instruction of the home health aide must be provided by a skilled professional such as an OTR, PT, or RN. Some agencies allow only the RN to supervise a home health aide and, in fact, this is the most common arrangement. It is important to check with an agency's individual policies for further clarification.

Home health aides are trained to take care of the patient and may often consider it their responsibility to do as much for the patient as possible. However, when occupational therapy services are being provided, the focus changes to encourage and train the patient to do as much for himself or herself as possible. The occupational therapy practitioner should collaborate with the aide and coordinate those components of the occupational therapy program that affect the aide's duties and responsibilities. The practitioner can enlist the cooperation of the aide in following through with certain aspects of the occupational therapy treatment program.

For example, if the aide is assisting the patient with bathing and dressing activities, the occupational therapy practitioner should instruct the aide in utilizing appropriate methods that would allow the patient to perform more independently. The aide can also be asked to monitor the patient's performance between occupational therapy visits. The use of checklists that outline the patient's requirements for assistance may also be useful tools in communicating to the aide the desired amount of help that should be given.

B. Certified Occupational Therapy Assistant

The COTA is supervised by the OTR. Supervision is an interactive process that requires both the COTA and the OTR to share responsibility. The OTR should provide supervision and the COTA should seek it. The degree and kind of supervision required will be dependent upon the experience level of the COTA, the establishment of service competency, and the complexity and stability of the patient population to be treated. Specific supervision requirements vary according to public health, state, and agency rules and regulations, and various standard setting organizations such as the Joint Commission on the Accreditation of Health Care Organizations (JCAHO) and Community Health Accreditation Programs, Inc. (CHAP). Although regulatory requirements for supervision may differ, the American Occupational Therapy Association (AOTA) recommends that COTAs, at all levels, receive general (at least monthly) direct contact with supervision available as needed (AOTA, 1993).

In supervising the COTA, the OTR should clearly outline and document a plan. The plan should describe the types and frequency of supervision to be used. Medicare may, on occasion, request to see the supervisory plan. The OTR and COTA should schedule joint visits according to the guidelines of the individual state regulatory board or Medicare. Telephone consultation and review of documentation offer other opportunities for supervisory contact. The occupational therapist is encouraged to read and countersign all notes written by the COTA and may be required to do so by some agencies and reimbursers. If a countersignature is required, it should be clearly stated as a requirement in the agency's policies, procedures, or protocols. Countersignature alone does not offer adequate supervision for the COTA nor does it replace other supervisory methods such as cotreatment and phone collaboration.

Occupational therapy practitioners should be aware of the fact that some private insurance companies, and some Medicaid programs, do not allow COTAs to treat patients. Medicare guidelines do specifically allow for COTA's to treat patients. A letter citing Medicare guidelines addressed to the administration of the program denying coverage for a COTA's services, may lead to reconsideration.

Billing joint visits to the home health agency, which would allow the OTR to conduct on-site supervision of the COTA, varies from agency to agency. In situations where agencies will not pay both practitioners for a joint visit, other alternatives need to be explored. For example, some agencies require that the OTR perform an on-site supervisory/treatment visit without the presence of a COTA. In this case, the OTR visits the patient and assesses his or her progress and outcome achievement in order to determine the COTA's effectiveness. After the visit, the OTR discusses the findings

with the COTA, offers feedback, and makes suggestions for adjustments in the treatment approach or activities. Another solution is for the OTR/COTA team to agree to split the fee for the supervisory visit. The OTR may also decide to provide supervision by conducting a supervisory visit with the COTA outside of the patient's home or by phone.

No matter what the option, the supervisory visit should be documented by both of the practitioners to ensure compliance with supervisory guidelines. Updated goals and treatment plans should be included in the documentation.

C. Occupational Therapist

The supervision of the OTR will vary greatly depending on if the therapist is an employee or an independent contractor. As an independent contractor, the OTR is his or her own supervisor. As an agency employee, the OTR will have a designated supervisor. A rehabilitation coordinator, nursing supervisor, or senior OTR may serve as a supervisor.

When a practitioner from another discipline serves as the occupational therapy supervisor, the supervision that is provided is more administrative in nature. The supervisor in these instances is not responsible for overseeing the therapist's clinical practice. It is recommended that when supervised by someone from another discipline, that access to appropriate clinical supervision and consultation be available to the therapist.

VIII. Conclusion

Teamwork is very important in the home health setting. Most patients are seen by at least two disciplines, and three or four is not uncommon. Coordination among disciplines is important to avoid confusion, overlap of services, and to promote consistency. Support of other disciplines in the treatment process also maximizes treatment outcomes. Without a commitment to teamwork and the necessary communication that accompanies it, treatment can become fragmented. The practitioner's dedication to both of these factors can ensure that the patient's treatment will be enhanced.

References

American Occupational Therapy Association. (1993). Occupational therapy roles. *American Journal of Occupational Therapy, 47*(12), 1087–1098.

American Occupational Therapy Association. (1987). Entry-level role delineation for registered occupational therapists (OTRs) and certified occupational therapy assistants (COTAs). *American Journal of Occupational Therapy, 41*, 798–803.

Chapter 4

Referral to Home Health Occupational Therapists

by Michael J. Steinhauer, OTR, MPH, FAOTA

with contributions from Karen Johnson, OTR

I. Introduction

A referral is the channel of communication through which cases are directed to a service provider; in this case a home health agency. This chapter presents an overview of the referral from initial sources to documentation. Unique strategies for increasing referrals to occupational therapy in home health are also discussed.

II. The Referral Process

Each agency has specific procedures and forms for handling referrals. Although procedures may vary by agency, many are common to most areas of home health practice (see Figure 1). Occupational therapy practitioners should become familiar with the procedures implemented by each agency for which they work. They will then be able to assess patients more effectively and in a timely and appropriate manner.

FIGURE 1. THE REFERRAL PROCESS.

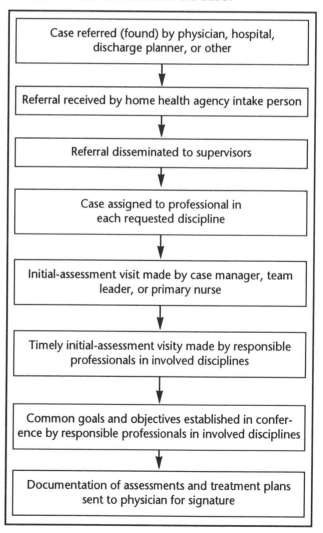

Case referred (found) by physician, hospital, discharge planner, or other

Referral received by home health agency intake person

Referral disseminated to supervisors

Case assigned to professional in each requested discipline

Initial-assessment visit made by case manager, team leader, or primary nurse

Timely initial-assessment visity made by responsible professionals in involved disciplines

Common goals and objectives established in conference by responsible professionals in involved disciplines

Documentation of assessments and treatment plans sent to physician for signature

III. Medicare Considerations

Under current Medicare law, occupational therapy is not deemed as a qualifying service for purposes of the Part A home health benefit. Thus, in Medicare-certified home health agencies, occupational therapists and occupational therapy assistants may treat patients only when a beneficiary requires the need of one of the qualifying services first. Examples of a qualifying service include nursing, physical therapy, or speech-language pathology. In addition the beneficiary must, under Medicare's definition, be homebound (see Chapter 1 for definition of "homebound" on page 3), and benefit from the intermittent services that Medicare reimburses. To comply with the qualifying regulation, some agencies designate an attending nurse as the case manager even though the patient may ultimately only require occupational therapy. When this occurs, the nurse may open the case with a nursing evaluation and a follow-up visit, but close the nursing portion of the case after making a referral for the occupational therapy practitioner to address continuing needs. When occupational therapy is included in the original plan of care, the service may continue and be recertified after all other professions have discharged the patient.

However, some fiscal intermediaries may not interpret Medicare regulations consistently. They may stipulate that when occupational therapy is not included in the original plan of care, it may continue only as long as a primary skilled service is also being provided. When and how long occupational therapy may continue depends on agency policy and the interpretation of Medicare regulations by the agency's fiscal intermediary. Typically, recertification is justified when a patient's homebound status is unchanged and he or she is making reasonable, measurable progress toward justifiable, functional, and useful goals.

After receiving a referral but before scheduling the initial visit, the occupational therapist confers with the case manager and other team members to assure the coordination of services. This helps to maximize care and clearly delineate the role of each team member. The occupational therapist should then contact the patient and his or her family to make an appointment.

The routing of a referral varies from agency to agency, so policy on the timeliness of the initial visit may differ. When the initial visit has been completed, the occupational therapist writes a summary of the evaluation, identifying the patient's problems and needs, while establishing a treatment plan. For Medicare and Medicaid (or the state's equivalent), this information must be recorded on specific forms and submitted to the referring physician for a signature. The forms should be completed according to the policies and procedures of the individual agency and its fiscal intermediary. For reimbursment sources other then Medicare or Medicaid, many agencies have developed their own baseline data forms. Some agencies have separate physician approval forms for each discipline while others use an integrated form.

IV. Sources of Referrals to Home Health Occupational Therapy

Referrals for home health come from a variety of sources. They may originate from acute care settings, physicians, registered nurses, physical therapists, patients themselves, speech-language pathologists, social workers, families, or community advocates. Other agencies providing patient care may make referrals to a home health agency such as rehabilitation centers, extended-care facilities, nursing homes, or community health care facilities (e.g., adult day-care centers, clinics, centers for the disabled).

In addition, agencies in another geographic area may refer patients. For example, suppose a patient received home health care in his or her home in another state. The patient requires further therapy and will still be homebound after relocating. The patient is referred to a home health agency in his or her new place of residence, and a physician is contacted there to assume responsibility for prescribing and signing orders for continued home health services.

Most typically, however, hospitals and skilled nursing facilities have discharge planners or social service departments that plan for a patient's return home. Some home health agencies hire individuals, often nurses or social workers, to go into hospitals or skilled nursing facilities to serve as discharge planners and perform case finding for the agency's catchment area. Before a patient leaves an institution, a discharge planner not only refers the patient to an appropriate agency, but also helps to organize a home health program. This process may include assessing the need for durable medical equipment, skilled nursing care, services of home health aides, and appropriate rehabilitation services. Ideally, the discharge planner would confer with the physician, floor nurses, rehabilitation staff, and the patient's family before arranging for any services or equipment to be provided.

V. Referral Assignment

In large home health agencies, referrals are usually received by an intake person who is often a nurse or a qualified secretary, if state regulations permit. This person gives copies of the referral to a case manager or supervisor. When the referral includes orders for occupational therapy, the case manager or the supervisor assigns the case to an appropriate occupational therapist or the rehabilitation supervisor.

In small agencies, a nurse, a therapist, or a secretary may receive the referral and forward it directly to the professional(s) who will be providing the requested services. Occupational therapists may receive the referral by phone, mail, or fax, or they may be expected to pick up the information at the agency. Routing depends on an agency's referral policies and procedures.

The determination of an appropriate assignment is based not only on caseload but also on special skills. Increasingly, pediatric and mental health patients are being treated at home so the demand for occupational therapists and occupational therapy assistants trained in these specialties is growing. When an agency receives a pediatric or mental health referral, the case should be assigned to a therapist who is skilled in those areas of practice. An agency with only a few specialists on staff may refer such cases to another agency whose staff has the requisite skills.

Another factor in appropriate referral assignment is geography. Some agencies divide their rehabilitation staff into teams that cover specified territories. These teams usually comprise nurses, physical therapists, occupational therapists, speech-language pathologists, social workers, and home health aides. A patient who lives within a certain area is assigned to the team with that particular geographic jurisdiction.

When a patient is being readmitted to an agency with an exacerbating or new medical problem that requires occupational therapy intervention, the supervisor should attempt to refer the patient to the occupational therapist who provided services during the previous admission. Reassignment to a familiar person provides good continuity of care and saves the time and energy required in establishing new relationships.

VI. Increasing Referrals

Strategies for increasing referrals to home health, and specifically to occupational therapy services, include the following (Kelly & Steinhauer, 1991):

- Make rounds with home health nurses.

- Provide in-service training to nursing field staff and intake coordinators through brief presentations at staff meetings. Utilize Health Care Financing Administration-designated (HCFA) treatment codes for occupational therapy. Supplement the in-service with consumer-oriented information from associations like the Arthritis Foundation, National Multiple Sclerosis Society, American Heart Association, and others, and health professional information sheets provided by the American Occupational Therapy Association (AOTA) such as *Occupational Therapy and Arthritis* and *When You Are Recovering from a Stroke.*

- Have lunch with the agency's marketing, public relations/community relations staff, and intake coordinators.

- Educate the agency staff network by participating in aide competency training sessions, student orientations, and care planning meetings. Some home health state associations have developed holiday greeting cards for patients that can include a short but meaningful message about the value of occupational therapy services.

- Review intake referrals and participate in agency-required clinical record review activities to find potential clients. Look for reports of dependence in activities of daily living (ADL), transfers, sensory losses, and other areas.

- Network with hospital-based occupational therapy practitioners regarding their patients that are ready for discharge. You can provide a home safety evaluation checklist for families to complete before discharge and have it reviewed by the occupational therapy practitioner for a possible occupational therapy referral to address problematic areas. You can also invite the hospital-based occupational therapy practitioner to spend a few hours with the home health occupational therapy practitioner so that each can gain a greater appreciation for the considerations of the workplace setting.

- Make every attempt to set up a "speaker's bureau" with other occupational therapy practitioners with expertise in particular areas. Ask to be invited to speak at support groups (e.g., arthritis, multiple sclerosis, stroke clubs), church groups, meal sites for the elderly, and senior citizen social clubs. Discuss adaptive equipment, and transfer and ADL techniques for the disabled. Referrals can easily be generated directly from these audiences. A slide/tape program can be developed for these kinds of sessions.

- Submit success stories about specific patient diagnostic groups to magazines, newspapers, and consumer health publications.

- When working with health maintenance organization (HMO) and insurance company personnel, try to make an appointment with their nursing or case management staff. Again, utilize the slide/tape program and the AOTA literature to get the point across.

- Local television and radio shows are almost always looking for program ideas and they should be approached without hesitation.

- Health fairs are also a common outlet for sharing the value of occupational therapy in home health with other providers and participants.

Many home health administrators will support activities designed to educate the community about the use of home health services that in turn will result in more referrals to the agency. Another positive point is that most of the activities described above do not require large expenditures for the agency. However, the primary issue for the occupational therapy practitioner may be that of seeking reimbursement for time spent working on these projects. This matter should be settled in advance of any work performed. Therapists who are in practice for themselves and who may contract with a group of home health agencies, may consider developing educational and marketing materials at their own cost, and then selling or renting the presentation on a per project basis to the agencies.

Medicare has very broad guidelines for reimbursement of these "advertising" costs. According to Jansak (1990), three tests that help measure the reimbursement potential of marketing costs are the Medium, the Distribution, and the Message. He suggests it is best to consider the following:

> Is the medium consistent with a distribution strategy that can be targeted to specific groups (usually allowable) or is the medium of a more general nature such as TV, radio, or newspaper advertising (usually not allowable)? Printed media are more likely to be found allowable such as brochures or magazines that can be circulated to the provider's patients and their families.
>
> Is the distribution confined to patients, employees, and state and county medical societies (usually allowable) or is it distributed to the general public (sometimes not allowable)?

Distribution aimed at people in the health care chain that "need to know" may be safe.

> Is the message intended to make people aware of the agency and its services—to present a good public image (usually allowable); present facts about the provider (allowable), or does the material "sell" the provider's services (usually not allowable)? The Provider Reimbursement Review Board (PRRB) has consistently held that public health messages are not allowable on the presumption that they are aimed at increasing use of services and not related to patient care. (p. 106)

VII. Referrals Appropriate to Occupational Therapy

The opportunities for appropriate and timely referrals will be greater the more closely occupational therapy practitioners confer and work with nurses, physical therapists, speech-language pathologists, social workers, and discharge planners. When a referral does not include a request for occupational therapy but such intervention appears to be appropriate, the nursing or rehabilitation supervisor may request a professional in another discipline to assess the need for such therapy. Consultation with an occupational therapist is useful in making this determination. If a need exists, the nurse, physical therapist, or speech-language pathologist who has made the initial evaluation, contacts the referring physician for additional orders to cover an occupational therapy evaluation and the case manager or the supervisor assigns the case to an occupational therapist. An alternate procedure in some agencies is to have an occupational therapist make an evaluation visit, obtaining prior physician approval as required by agency policy. The occupational therapist then contacts the physician for additional orders to cover further evaluation and treatments.

Periodic in-service programs conducted by occupational therapy practitioners concerning their role in home health can assist supervisors and other professional staff in recognizing their patient's need for occupational therapy services. These programs should emphasize early and timely intervention so that patients are given the opportunity to regain independent function; not simply learn substitute compensation skills.

The occupational therapy practitioner who works in a home health agency should be familiar with all of the agency's home health programs or specialties like support services and mental health programs, and evaluate them as potential referral sources. Familiarity with community organizations and contact with their staff both formally and informally enable the occupational therapy practitioner to enhance his or her program and to refer patients back to the community after treatment. This contact also educates social service personnel in the community about services that occupational therapy can provide. Some commonly used resources are the Commission for the Blind, the Easter Seal Society, and the Division of Vocational Rehabilitation.

Ideally, practitioners working for a home health agency are available to serve on professional agency advisory boards and utilization review committees. In addition, occupational therapists and occupational therapy assistants should participate in case record review committees and rehabilitation team conferences. The visibility and the input from each professional representing the perspective of his or her discipline assists an agency in providing the most effective, appropriate, and timely treatment.

Information packets prepared and distributed to referral sources (i.e., individual physicians, hospitals, skilled nursing facilities) by an agency, also help physicians prescribe the most appropriate therapy intervention when referring patients to a home health agency. Such packets might describe the types of services provided by the various disciplines and list the diagnoses that will benefit from them. A list of diagnoses for which occupational therapy is frequently requested also serves to alert intake personnel to order an occupational therapy evaluation on the initial referral form. A sample list of diagnoses follows. It is taken from the revised *Guidelines for Utilization of Specialized Rehabilitation Services in Home Health Agencies* (Home Health Agency Assembly, 1985):

> Referral for occupational therapy services is appropriate for those individuals with motor, sensory, cognitive, perceptual, emotional, or social deficits associated with, but not limited to, the following diagnostic categories:
>
> • Congenital or acquired neurological deficits
>
> • Developmental delay
>
> • Neuropathies
>
> • Head trauma
>
> • Paraplegia
>
> • Quadriplegia
>
> • Cerebral vascular accident
>
> • Cardiac disease or disorder

• Respiratory disease

• Fractures

• Osteo- or rheumatoid arthritis

• Collagen disorders

• Joint replacement

• Amputation

• Visual disorder

• Psychological disorder (e.g., depression, schizophrenia) (Section V)

Although the examples above delineate a medical model, social factors should also be considered as potential benchmarks for a possible referral to occupational therapy. For instance, a patient returning home alone may have a more intense need for occupational therapy services to evaluate and provide training and instruction to use adaptive equipment than for another patient who may rely on family caregiver support to accomplish ADL.

Having one of the above diagnoses does not in and of itself indicate a need for referral. An unexplained loss of function or inability to cope with tasks of daily living, combined with a potential for improvement, are additional criteria for referral. Another example of referral guidelines for consumers and physicians is the AOTA information literature, *Occupational Therapy Is Important When You Are in Need of Home Health Services* (see Appendix B).

VIII. Referral Information

Typically, a referral to occupational therapy services in a home health agency is received one of two ways. The first common possibility, as discussed earlier, comes from the original referral source who referred the patient to home health to initiate services. For example, a discharge planner in a hospital may refer the patient to a home health agency and the discharge planner would then indicate what services are generally needed or should be ordered. An example of a generic home health agency referral form can be found in Appendix C. In this case, the agency-level referral form is the most typical document used to initiate occupational therapy services. The request for occupational therapy is generally a broad one with unspecific goals and orders.

The other most common avenue for a referral to occupational therapy in home health comes from a home health team member who has already been seeing the patient and has identified a need for occupational therapy. In this latter case, it is a good idea for the occupational therapist and occupational therapy assistant to develop a referral form specific to their program. The purpose of such a form is to cue other team members to the unique contribution that occupational therapy can offer and encourages questions about specific concerns that can be addressed by the occupational therapy practitioners.

Recognizing that there will be overlap between what might be required on a referral form to initiate any service, and those elements that comprise a good occupational therapy-specific referral form, the following elements are guidelines for inclusion:

The patient:

- Patient's name, address, telephone number, and date of birth.
- If there is no phone, how may the patient be contacted (e.g., through a relative or a neighbor, or by going directly to the patient's home)?
- Who should be contacted if the patient is unable to reach a telephone or speak on it, or does not speak English?
- The patient's primary language, and is anyone available to interpret?
- Family's name, address and telephone number.
- Instructions for entry (e.g., "Use side door" or "Call 15 minutes before visit so door may be opened").

Referring physician:

- Referring physician, or patient's physician if referral is from another source.
- Physician's name, address, and telephone number.

Primary diagnosis:

- Diagnosis for which agency care is requested.
- Date of onset.
- Dates of hospital stays if the patient has been admitted for treatment.

Secondary diagnoses (other medical and physical problems) with dates of onset that:

- Affect the patient's ability to function.
- Validate the need for service at home.
- Confirm the patient's homebound status (see "Conditions for Coverage of Home Health Services," Appendix D).

Medications:

- Medications the patient is taking including doses and frequency.
- Special diet that the patient must follow.
- Any allergies the patient has.
- Name and telephone number of the patient's pharmacy.

Payment source:

- How the patient's care is being reimbursed—Medicare, Medicaid, major medical coverage, private insurance, United Way (or its local equivalent), municipal health funds, agency "free care," self-pay, or other.
- Visit limits imposed by a third-party payer.

Date for start of service:

- Date referral source wants each specific service to begin. A nursing visit and an evaluation of the need for a home health aide may be necessary before or immediately after the patient's return home.

Services, frequency of visits, and duration:

- Disciplines that are to provide services to the patient, how often, and for how long.
- In some agencies, this is left to the judgment of the nurse and the therapists—what therapeutic interventions (e.g., training in skills of daily living, orthotics, or passive range of motion) will be needed?
- Treatment is often determined by the nurse or the therapist after the evaluation visit.

Contraindications or precautions (conditions that may limit treatment) for example:

- Weight-bearing tolerances.
- Cardiac and respiratory problems.
- Seizures.

Information about the referral source:

- Person making the referral (other than the patient's physician).
- Source of the referral.
- Relationship of referring individual to patient.
- Conditions on which referral source is judging patient's need for home health.
- Patient's level of function before onset of the illness or the disability.
- Homebound status—is the patient able to leave the house with ease, or is maximum assistance required? Is he or she bedbound?

The family:
- Who is in the home to assist the patient?
- Does the patient live alone?
- Does the patient have a home health aide?
- Who are the patient's "significant others" (people who are important to his or her care and well-being)?
- What are the directions to get to the patient's home?

Some agencies prefer referral forms that are used to initiate multiple services but the information provided is general and offers limited information to the providers of the requested services. Requests for services may also be vague or incomplete. Ideally, cues are included on the form to encourage more specific orders than simply "evaluate and treat as needed."

After the team member who opens the case makes the initial evaluation visit, he or she may determine a need for further treatment or service. At this time, an ancillary referral form is used that supplements the original with orders for the additional treatments or services. This form may be written following a call to the physician for verbal orders, and then sent to him or her for a signature. Ancillary referral forms should include:
- Patient ID number
- Date the referral was made.
- Clinical facts supporting the need for additional services.
- Patient's prior level of function.
- Services requested.
- Recommended procedures .
- Frequency and duration.
- Projected goals.

The forms should also include the name of the person requesting the additional orders. When a nurse or other professional requests additional physician's orders for an occupational therapy evaluation, the occupational therapist should make the evaluation and submit the treatment plan and supplementary order form to the physician. This form, when signed, covers further occupational therapy visits.

After each discipline has made an initial visit, the name of the case manager and each of the service providers should be listed on the intake sheet or the referral form. This information is a resource for contacting other professionals working with the patient as well as for scheduling and coordinating the plan of care, and setting common goals. Including directions to the patient's home in his or her chart facilitates provision of services by all professionals.

IX. Timeliness of Referrals

Diagnosis-related groups (DRGs) influence the length of hospital stays based on diagnosis, age, date of onset, and other criteria affecting referrals to home health. As a result, patients appear to be returning home earlier more acutely ill, less medically stable, and less able to tolerate treatment than in previous years. Another trend is the reduction in the length of treatment. To provide the best plan of care for this type of patient, the primary nurse or the case manager may make an evaluation and, in consultation with the occupational therapist, determine when occupational therapy treatment should begin. The occupational therapist should make the professional judgment on the timeliness and the appropriateness of treatment. If the therapist considers occupational therapy to be inappropriate at the time, he or she should contact the physician and discuss delaying the start of treatment until the patient is physically able to participate. The therapist should inform the physician of the results of the occupational therapy evaluation and project a date for therapy to start.

Some third-party payers require that a nurse see a patient within 48 hours of when an agency receives a referral. Agencies, therefore, try to make the initial patient contact within that period. An agency's policy may state that all appropriate professionals must see or talk by telephone with a patient within a specific time frame. To be in compliance, the occupational therapist should know and follow the policies and procedures of the agency and reimbursement sources regarding the initial visit. It is helpful to be familiar with the time limits set by insurance payers as well as by Medicare.

After making the initial evaluation visit the case manager, who most commonly is designated by agency policy as the nurse or physical therapist, may call the physician to request additional services such as occupational therapy. The initial evaluation visit often provides additional medical and psychosocial data not included in the original referral. This information may be helpful to the occupational therapist in planning and scheduling his or her initial visit. For example, the evaluation visit may offer information such as the following: "Patient lethargy not conducive to therapy at this time", or "No one in home to open door after 1:00 p.m."

If the occupational therapist is unable to make an initial visit within the agency's time frame for reasons other than the patient's condition, he or she should contact the patient or the family to schedule the visit as soon as possible. A note recording this contact, the reason for the delay in providing service, and the proposed date for the initial visit should be included in the patient's chart.

By contacting the patient's home when the referral is first received and by documenting this action, the occupational therapist is in compliance with most third- party regulations. A late referral to occupational therapy or a delayed initial visit may make goals, which may have been attainable with earlier intervention, unrealistic in the time remaining for treatment of the patient.

X. Physician's Prescriptions

When a physician refers a patient to an agency for a specific medical problem that is not appropriate for occupational therapy treatment but it is later determined that the patient requires occupational therapy for another diagnosis, a second physician may have to sign the orders. For example, suppose a patient who has been hospitalized for a graft to an ulceration on a leg also has a history of rheumatoid arthritis. Following her discharge from the hospital, the patient has an exacerbation of the rheumatoid arthritis. She is unable to care for herself or leave home without maximum assistance. The surgeon's referral for home health services specifies: "Nursing daily to change dressings and observe wound site." The nurse requests a referral for an occupational therapy evaluation and treatment: "Patient homebound because of draining wound. Exacerbation of RA and dependent in all ADLs."

The orders for occupational therapy are sent for a signature to the physician who cares for the patient's general health problems and/or her arthritis. A copy of the orders is sent to the surgeon who is treating the ulcer for his or her information.

Occupational therapists and occupational therapy assistants should retain a copy of the signed physician's orders for their own records. When an agency does not receive signed orders within a reasonable period (set by applicable state law and agency policy and procedure), the physician is contacted and duplicate orders are sent for his or her signature. Most agencies have a policy to cover a physician's noncompliance. However, in most of these types of cases, the care would have to be terminated unless it is authorized by a physician's signed orders.

When a physician requests a service that the occupational therapist regards as inappropriate for a particular patient, the therapist is responsible for contacting the physician and discussing the problem. Usually, clarification of occupational therapy treatment resolves the situation. If it does not, the therapist should request help from his or her agency supervisor. Utilization Review Committees or Peer Review Committees within the agency may also provide support in handling an inappropriate referral. State occupational therapy associations are often able to help an occupational therapist or an occupational therapy assistant deal with problems regarding practice. Further, AOTA's Practice and Government Relations Departments will assist occupational therapy practitioners in obtaining information to clarify their roles and services in relation to physicians and patients.

XI. Conclusion

In conclusion, referral is the basis for the caseload of the home health occupational therapist and occupational therapy assistant. It is evident that many strategies exist for finding cases. Referral information includes many elements that will guide the practitioner to designing meaningful treatment programs. If referral procedures within an agency limit or prevent adequate provision of occupational therapy treatment, the problem should be discussed with agency personnel in charge of handling referrals. Organized referral procedures should facilitate timely, appropriate, and effective occupational therapy treatment to every patient.

References

American Occupational Therapy Association. (1995). *Occupational therapy is important...When you are in need of home health services.* [Information sheet]. Bethesda, MD: Author.

Home Health Agency Assembly in New Jersey. (1985). *Guidelines for utilization of specialized rehabilitation services in home health agencies* (rev.ed.). Princeton, NJ: Author.

Jansak, J. (1990). Medicare Part A provider advertising costs: Are they allowable? *Home Health Line, 15,* 97–108.

Kelly, P.A., & Steinhauer, M.J. (1991). Strategies for increasing referrals for occupational therapy in home health care. *American Journal of Occupational Therapy, 45*(7), 656–658.

Chapter 5

Clinical Considerations for the Treatment of Patients With Physical Disabilities in Home Health

by Rebecca Austill-Clausen, MS, OTR, FAOTA

with contributions from Theodosia T. Kelsey, OTR, FAOTA

I. Introduction

Providing patients with occupational therapy in their own home environment is an extremely effective way to maximize their independence. Home-based occupational therapy is a natural extension of our profession's versatility and training in adaptive techniques, designed to enable patients to become functional and independent in their home.

The first four chapters of these guidelines addressed the home health care culture. This chapter will be more specific and concentrate on unique home health clinical considerations when working with patients who have physical disabilities.

II. Treatment Prioritization

Home health has changed radically in the last decade. Patients are being discharged from hospitals sicker and quicker than in the past ("GAO Study", 1985). The acute effects of problems caused by illness, disease, or injury may still remain upon hospital discharge. An intensive level of care in the home can be required, but a reliable support system may not be in place since adult family members may be unavailable or working during the day.

When patients return home, often their spouse, a significant other, or a home health aide may want to help them groom, bathe, and dress even if the individuals accomplished these activities independently in the hospital or rehabilitation center. Family cooperation can be stimulated by explaining why it is so important for patients to determine their own level of independence, rather than having others accomplish activities for them. Family stress may be relieved when the family understands that helping individuals work towards functional independence can facilitate safe and successful living without the need for further assistance.

Written instructions should be provided to home health aides and family members on ways to facilitate independence through proper positioning, cuing, and reasonable expectations within time constraints. Cooperation can be enhanced by involving the patient and the family in constructing the instructions, thus helping secure their commitment to the program's success.

Therapy is sometimes time-limited by reimbursement requirements. Thus, it may be necessary to select problems that have the best potential for resolution within a limited time frame. In addressing patient desires and needs in addition to the family's concerns as part of the occupational therapy program, priorities should be justifiable, measurable, and quantitative, and the outcomes need to validate the program.

Home-based treatment encourages patients receiving services to work in concert with the occupational therapy practitioner to determine their own goals. Occupational therapists with contributions from occupational therapy assistants are skilled in evaluating the patient's cultural, sociological, physical, cognitive, sensorimotor, and psychosocial areas to help determine the most functional method for completing an activity in the home environment. The skilled occupational therapy practitioner works with the patient and family to help determine who is the most appropriate person to complete the activity, whether it be the individual receiving services or the family members. In home health, the family may be the "recipient" of service, rather than just the patient. There is a tremendous amount of family interaction in home health treatment, since the family is usually present when occupational therapy is being provided.

It is important for the home health occupational therapy practitioner to concentrate on issues that will help alleviate the patient's dependence at home. Occupational therapy treatment priorities should address issues that help the patient and the family become independent and safe in their own home environment.

III. Evaluation

Occupational therapy evaluation in the home is considerably different than an occupational therapy evaluation in the clinic. A variety of factors cannot be controlled, yet must be dealt with on an immediate and individual basis. These factors may include the environmental setting, ethnic diversity, limited work space, and the presence of family members during the evaluation, which while necessary, may be distracting to both the occupational therapy practitioner and the individual receiving services. If an occupational therapy assistant is involved, the occupational therapist is expected to collaborate with the assistant as appropriate during the evaluation and treatment of the patient.

The practitioner might use the initial 5 to 10 minutes of the evaluation to comment positively on the patient's home environment, the patient's abilities that are observed immediately, or the community in general. This rapport breaks the ice and gains the attention of the individual receiving services, and the family. A few insightful, open-ended questions that encourage participation by those present can facilitate this interaction.

Evaluation of the overall home situation, followed by an evaluation of variables specific to treatment in the home, will be ongoing and may change as the occupational therapy practitioner gains familiarity with the patient, his or her cultural environment, specific abilities, therapeutic priorities, and family expectations. A definition of the patient's previous level of function, both from the patient and the family members, is important in setting long-term goals. A comparison of the patient's report of his or her abilities, combined with the family's report and the discharge information generated from the referring agency, all need to be evaluated to provide the most appropriate goals. The family may feel that the mediation of certain problems has more immediacy than others. The family's priorities, in concert with the patient's and the practitioner's priorities, should all be factored into the treatment plan.

Often the initial evaluation visit generally acquaints the occupational therapist with the patient, caregivers, and the actual physical environment in which he or she will have to work. Subsequent visits may more clearly define patient strengths and deficits. On the initial evaluation visit, there may be a need to address multiple procedures, or be limited to a specific problem determined by the patient and the therapist (e.g., a caregiver who is unable to transfer the patient to the commode). In addressing this one need, the practitioner will have a chance to observe the patient's ability to participate and the abilities of the designated caregiver to safely assist and work with the patient. Subsequent visits following the initial evaluation may encompass (but not be limited to) in-depth evaluation and treatment of the following areas: environmental safety needs; motor coordination; activities of daily living (ADL) skills; sensory, perceptual, and cognitive abilities; a need for splints; and leisure activities. Subsequent visits may also include an evaluation of architectural barriers and durable medical equipment (DME). Each of these areas is discussed in this chapter. The discussion is not intended to be comprehensive but to stimulate thought, direction, and creativity for occupational therapy evaluation and treatment in the home health arena.

Appendix E contains a sample form used in an occupational therapy evaluation for a Medicare-certified home health agency.

IV. Evaluation and Treatment Areas

A. Environmental Safety Needs

The fundamental role of the occupational therapy practitioner is to treat and teach functional safety in the home. In the home health setting, environmental safety needs include functional communication and emergency response mechanisms, along with home management safety procedures. Table 1 demonstrates a few guidelines for these criteria in the home.

Patient safety also includes signs of negligence or abuse. In today's high stress environment, the physically demanding or care-intensive patient in the home has the potential to provoke behaviors seen less frequently 10 years ago. Sometimes the signs are subtle and need to be pursued to determine whether the patient has indeed been mistreated physically and emotionally. Whenever there is a suspicion of untoward action involving a patient, it should be reported to the home health team manager as well as to others who are treating the patient. This process enables each person to be aware of a potentially dangerous situation.

B. Motor Coordination

The patient's functional mobility affects their environmental safety and is therefore a high priority for the initial evaluation, ongoing treatment, and family training. In the home, evaluation of gross and fine motor coordination, and dexterity is often evaluated within the context of functional skills. Ambulation, balance, control of wheelchair (if used), and transfer skills are usually observed during the initial visit as the patient moves throughout the home. Evaluating finger dexterity,

Evaluation Areas	Treatment Ideas
Functional communication: Dialing telephone	Preprogrammed, automatic memory-dialer telephone with push-button emergency numbers.
Telephone location	Make accessible to bedroom, kitchen, and living room.
Emergency communication	Portable phone to carry in pocket or in walker bag. Push button emergency "Medic-Alert" systems, worn around neck or as a bracelet, to alert hospital and/or ambulance.
Unable to speak	Use of TDD (telecommunication device for the deaf). Use of word or picture board.
Lighting	Encourage high wattage bulbs (75–100 watts) to increase visibility.
Gas stove	Discourage use of pilot light for heat due to unsafe gas seepage.

TABLE 1. ENVIRONMENTAL SAFETY IN THE HOME.

coordination, and handwriting skills are important functional activities to address and treat.

Table 2 (see p. 32) is not intended to be an exhaustive list of gross and fine motor coordination and dexterity skills, but is presented to stimulate thought about these areas specifically for the home health occupational therapy practitioner.

Naturally, a full motor evaluation also includes lateral and bilateral integration elements, and an evaluation of praxis, visual motor integration, and oral motor control. A further delineation of sensorimotor components addresses sensory awareness, sensory awareness and processing areas. A neuromusculoskeletal evaluation in the home includes range of motion measurements, muscle tone, strength, endurance, reflexes, postural control, and postural alignment to help complete the home health practitioners understanding of the patient's functional motor skills.

C. Sensory

A patient's sensory awareness and sensory processing abilities are essential areas to be evaluated

Evaluation Areas	Evaluation and Treatment Ideas
Functional mobility	Observe patient ambulating to various rooms to assess balance, endurance, fatigue, and supervision needs.
Transfer ability	Observe patient transferring to/from sofa, bed, kitchen and living room chairs, toilet seats, etc.
Object manipulation	Have patient manipulate kitchen utensils, including removal/replacement from drawers.
	Have patient remove refrigerator items and transport them to counter/table.
	Observe patient handling grooming articles, evaluate location, closeness to mirror, etc.
Writing skills	Evaluate patient's ability to write checks; suggest sending bank sample of patient's "new" signature since patient incurred disability.
	Observe patient preparing kitchen lists.
	Have patient prepare schedule of therapy visits.

TABLE 2. MOTOR COORDINATION.

and treated in home health, especially for the patient living alone. Awareness of sensory deficits is important for problems of neglect such as poor arm position during wheelchair use or ambulation, handling of hot beverages and food, arm stabilization during transfers, and zipping of clothing. A home health occupational therapy practitioner needs to teach the patient with olfactory deficits how to examine and observe "old" food in the refrigerator, since the patient cannot smell rancid food. Adequate illumination may reduce what appears to be a visual problem. Teaching the patient to be aware of sensory deficiencies is particularly important for bathing, kitchen safety, ironing, and meal preparation activities.

D. Perception

Evaluating and treating perceptual processing abilities is imperative for effective home treatment particularly in regards to ADL skills and instrumental activities of daily living (IADL). Working

on body scheme, right-left discrimination, and depth perception can all be effectively addressed during dressing training in the patient's bedroom, training for meal preparation, and self-feeding. Walking the patient through his home or around a room may pinpoint problems with visual neglect, topographical orientation, spatial relations, eye/hand coordination, and figure ground. The individual who steps high to clear a flower in the pattern of their rug may need further testing of his or her perceptual processing abilities.

In many homes today, interactive video and computer games are available. This is especially true in homes where there are young people. The practitioner might want to consider using some of the games that require eye/hand coordination, tracking skills, visual spatial awareness, and dexterity. These games can also work on cognitive integration skills including attention span, memory, problem solving, sequencing, and categorization. Often, because these activities are not so "therapeutically" apparent, the patient will keep working at this task for an extended period of time.

E. Cognition

Evaluation of an individual's alertness, distractibility, and orientation to date, time, and place can offer insights into his or her memory skills, attention span, and problem-solving abilities. Judgment and safety factors such as reliability in following procedures, impulsiveness, recognition of hazards, and the ability to call for help (telephone use) should always be considered, particularly if the patient is left alone for any period of time. In home health, individuals may have emergency response system devices or adapted phones with special buttons to press in case of emergencies (see previous section in this chapter on environmental safety needs). The patient's cognitive awareness regarding the use of these aids, along with their physical capability to use them, should be part of the cognitive and judgment skills evaluation and treatment. The occupational therapy practitioner should help the family plan for emergencies, when the patient is expected to be responsible for summoning help, by evaluating the patient's problem-solving abilities.

F. Activities of Daily Living (ADL)

Evaluating and treating ADL skills are essential components of providing occupational therapy in the home. The home health practitioner has the advantage of observing the patient in their own home environment. This enables the therapist to immediately evaluate the patient's safety, functional abilities, mobility, orientation, perception, specific daily living skills, and architectural barriers present during the completion of daily living tasks. The therapist should have the patient demonstrate his or her methods in managing routines of daily living because verbal reporting may camouflage safety, motivation, and energy problems.

With the more involved or bedbound patient, evaluating ADL concentrates on the patient's awareness of his or her own deficits, coping skills, and functional abilities (i.e., if the patient does not roll over to look at the therapist during the evaluation, is it because the patient is unaware of the therapist, unable to look at the therapist, or not interested in participating in therapy?) Working with the patient and his or her family on techniques to increase daily living independence, even if the patient is bedbound, can help maximize the patient's rehabilitation in their own home environment.

Consider the following categories of activity.

Toileting: Most occupational therapy practitioners working in the home do not use standardized assessment tools but can gain a wealth of information from basic activity analysis instead. Analyzing a patient's ability to role play the act of toileting can provide the home health practitioner with tremendous practical information. Asking the patient to go into the bathroom provides knowledge about functional mobility, ambulation, balance, and coordination. The practitioner learns about the patient's strength, endurance, and energy conservation techniques. Asking the patient to sit on the toilet provides data on positioning and transfer skills, problem solving, and cognitive awareness. Having the patient role play the act of removing clothes and wiping oneself can facilitate information on finger dexterity, bilateral integration, dressing abilities, zipping and buttoning skills, visual ability, and communication. Any problems noted during this initial role playing exercise require an actual observation of the patient's skills. Yet, this simple activity analysis can provide the home health occupational therapy practitioner with a tremendous amount of functional information critically important to the patient's safety in their own home.

Dressing: In the home, evaluating and treating dressing skills often becomes a major focus of the treatment program. It is important to consider the most appropriate place to teach dressing skills. Moving a dining room chair (with or without arms) to the bedroom, or having the patient sit on a commode placed in the bedroom may provide

Problem	Possible Solutions
Utensil width too small	Wrap handle with rubber grip tape, foam rubber, lightweight soft foam hair curler, rubber bands, splinting material, masking tape.
Plate/bowl slipping	Place damp towel under plate. Use Dycem (or less expensive nonskid material placed under rugs) under plate/bowl.
Food slipping	Use pie pan, lipped plate, plate guard.
Mugs/cups too heavy	Use lightweight commuter cups with large handles and removable lids.
Unable to reach mouth	Use long-handled iced tea spoon (often needs built-up handle).
Difficulty seeing plate/food	Use bright placemats. Place food in a variety of positions on plate to assess and maximize visual impact.
Inadequate lighting	Increase wattage of kitchen bulbs.

TABLE 3. LOW-COST MEALTIME ADAPTATIONS.

increased patient stability during dressing training. The patient's ability to select, gather, and carry his or her clothing from the floor, closets, and bureaus should be evaluated along with active dressing skills. Sometimes a change in routine from dressing on rising, to dressing after breakfast or after a bath can reduce stress, save energy, and ease family burdens if the initial dressing routine is inconvenient or time consuming.

Eating: Many patients can be independent in the basic skill of feeding themselves. Frequently the patient who may appear to require feeding assistance is independent when appropriate seating and adaptive equipment is used. Occupational therapy practitioners need to be aware of low-cost mealtime adaptations and techniques that can benefit the homebound patient (see Table 3).

G. Instrumental Activities of Daily Living (IADL)

IADL are described as complex daily living activities such as housework, meal preparation, cleaning, shopping, laundry, and cooking. In contrast, ADL have been categorized as activities required for self-maintenance such as dressing, bathing, and toileting (Hopkins & Smith, 1993; Pepper Commission, 1990; Law, 1992).

IADL are appropriate to evaluate, and may be appropriate to treat in the home health environment, depending on the patient's diagnosis, treatment priorities, and situation. Addressing a patient's ability to complete IADL is particularly important for high-functioning individuals and patients living alone. It is important that the home health practitioner be aware of how the patient implements these activities between visits, since some patients tend to overestimate their abilities. Money management, shopping, household maintenance, and community access are also appropriate to address in treatment, yet careful documentation of continued homebound status is imperative.

H. Leisure Routines

Leisure routines are an important aspect of home health. Occupational therapists and occupational therapy assistants can be reimbursed by Medicare for one to two visits for leisure evaluation and program planning (Health Care Financing Administration, 1986). Reimbursement for developing a leisure-based program depends on a home health agency's policy and the fiscal intermediary's interpretation. It is therefore highly recommended that other activities, particularly ones involving ADL skills, occur during a treatment session focusing on leisure routines. If an activity has a physical component (e.g., development of arm placement, pinch, grasp, or coordination through the use of board games), the practitioner should document both the physical and leisure components of the activity.

Leisure activities such as playing cards, checkers, handicrafts, sewing, woodworking, video or computer games, working on puzzles, reading, talking on the telephone, writing letters, and watching television can all be extremely important to help stimulate an individual's cognitive awareness and perceptual processing abilities. It is important to ask the family and the patient what leisure activities they engaged in prior to their illness. The occupational therapy practitioner can then adapt the leisure routine to fit the needs of the individual receiving service. A creative occupational therapy practitioner will find ways to incorporate components of the patient's preferred leisure time activities into his or her occupational therapy program.

Leisure time can include aspects of driving. Thus, another area to be addressed by the occupa-

tional therapy practitioner in home health is the ability to transfer into a car, which is particularly relevant when patients visit their doctor. Using household furniture to simulate car seat transfers, "talking" the individual through the car transfer process, and having the patient demonstrate their ability to enter the car as a passenger are all important variables. As individuals transition to outpatient status, they may be referred to a driving center for a driving evaluation. Contact with centers that give predriving assessment tests may help the occupational therapy practitioner focus on the skills most relevant to facilitating predriving training. The home health occupational therapy practitioner may find it useful to contact their state's Department of Transportation to learn about rules and regulations regarding their specific patient's needs. The occupational therapy practitioner needs to document very carefully the reason car transfer training and predriving activities are incorporated into treatment, since such activities could indicate that the patient is no longer homebound.

V. Interventions

A. Splints

Occasionally, the occupational therapist is asked to evaluate a patient's need for a splint. For reimbursement purposes, it is recommended that a physician's order be obtained before ordering or making such a splint. On occasion, a prefabricated hand splint can be ordered to fit the needs of the patient in the home. It is important that the occupational therapist check the fit, evaluate for pressure points, make minor adaptations, and instruct the patient, home health aide, and family in the application and wearing of the splint. Directions on the duration and frequency of use should be written out by the occupational therapy practitioners and placed in a highly visible location, such as above the patient's bed or on the refrigerator door.

B. Medication

The patient's ability to manage medication and self-administer insulin is an important area to evaluate, from a cognitive and a motoric standpoint. If the patient is mentally alert but physically unable to open their medication bottles, his or her pharmacist can be asked to discontinue use of child-proof containers. Weekly medication pill boxes are available from pharmacies to help organize medication schedules. The patient can also be asked to help write out their medication schedules, and check off on a list when it has been taken.

Home health occupational therapy practitioners need to be aware when the patient is taking a number of medications that, separately or combined, have the potential to cause side effects that could impact on their rehabilitation performance. If occupational therapy is the last remaining service in a home health situation, it is the practitioners responsibility to be observant of medication schedules, be alert as to whether the individual is actually taking their medication, note any medication problems, and report them immediately to the home health nurse or referring physician.

VI. Architectural Barriers and Durable Medical Equipment (DME)

An area of great need, which is specific to the occupational therapy practitioner working in home health, is the evaluation of architectural barriers and durable medical equipment (DME) requirements. If a patient has been discharged from an acute care hospital or a rehabilitation center, DME may already have been ordered (e.g., raised toilet seat, wheelchair, or toilet safety rails). Frequently the patient will need to be retrained on the proper procedures for safe use of the equipment in their own unique environment. Height, position, ease of transfer, and accessibility of equipment all need to be evaluated in the home, even though the occupational therapy practitioner has been informed that the patient was instructed in the hospital or rehabilitation center. If the equipment does not meet the patient's needs or is inappropriate for his or her home, the occupational therapy practitioner should inform the purchaser and ask for an exchange. Once the equipment has been used, it usually cannot be returned. Yet, equipment can be frequently obtained on a trial basis from a medical equipment supplier to assess patient suitability. The home health occupational therapy practitioner needs to know what DME will be covered by the patient's insurance or funding source, and what alternatives within the home might be suggested in order to provide the most appropriate equipment recommendations to the patient and the family.

Every room in the home presents obstacles for individuals using a wheelchair, walker, cane, or who have visual or perceptual impairments. In many cases, the occupational therapy practitioner may recognize a need to change the environment if the patient is to function independently or more effectively. However, the patient or others in the household, may want things to remain just the same. Communicating the patient's needs to the family members, along with suggestions which may only be temporary or change the general physical appearance as little as possible, may help facilitate agreement.

A. Bathroom Access and Use

The bathroom is one of the most important areas to evaluate completely for architectural barriers, safety, and the patient's independence since barriers usually exist in this area. The bathroom is often the smallest room in the home with the narrowest door. Therefore, the patient must employ more physical, visual, and functional skills to move within the bathroom environment. Patients who have been trained in bathroom independence in the hospital or rehabilitation center may be unable to translate these skills back to their own environment. Home health occupational therapists and occupational therapy assistants have a unique role to play in maximizing bathroom independence (see Tables 4–6 on pp. 36–37).

Toileting and bathing aids are not frequently reimbursed by Medicare or Medicaid. In some instances, private insurance companies will pay for this equipment, although payment often takes from 2 to 4 months and usually requires a physician's prescription. Community resources such as the Multiple Sclerosis Society, the Arthritis Foundation, church or community loan closets, senior citizens centers, the National Association of American Business Clubs, or home health agency loaner equipment may also be viable sources, depending upon an individual's diagnosis and situation.

B. Kitchen Access and Use

The kitchen is often filled with architectural barriers. A variety of low-cost solutions can facilitate functional independence in the kitchen. The following table is presented to stimulate thought, and is not intended to be an exhaustive list of kitchen adaptations (see Table 7 on p. 38).

The occupational therapy practitioner can suggest that patients do a mental inventory of what they need at each meal of the day to help stimulate memory and facilitate energy conservation principles. Items used most frequently should be stored near the front of and on lower shelves.

While many adapted kitchen tools are available through various suppliers of home medical equipment, using the individual's own tools with simple adaptations may fulfill the need and reduce the expense of purchasing yet another "gadget." Items that practitioners think might help, but do not really meet the individual's needs, become "gadgets." Anything that enables the individual to perform a task with minimal exertion, greater success, and in less time is a "tool." Some of the more commonly used items that often serve as tools are

Problem	Possible Solutions
Difficulty transferring to/from toilet	Toilet safety rails with armrests attached to back of toilet. Floor-mounted toilet safety rails. Floor-to-ceiling vertical rod with or without handle. Wall-mounted grab bars. 5" utility handles (door pulls) can be an inexpensive substitute for grab bars and installed on door frames or bathroom window sills. ***Caution:** Advise patients not to use towel racks, toilet paper dispensers, or wall-mounted sinks due to the equipment's questionable stability for transfer use.
Toilet too low	Raised toilet seats.
Need for grab bars and higher toilet	Commode without back placed over seat often called "3 in 1 commode" (has three uses as a commode, raised toilet seat, and bathtub bench); can adjust leg height and use commode arms as toilet armrests.
Unable to enter bathroom, or lacks the speed needed to reach toilet.	Use a portable commode, placed in the most accessible location.
Unable to reach toilet paper	Toilet paper holders: 1) Obtain holder to attach toilet paper to commode legs (available from local home medical equipment dealers) 2) Make toilet paper holder attachment from split coat hanger.

TABLE 4. TOILETING BARRIERS AND ADAPTATIONS.

Portable

Advantages	Disadvantages
Lightweight.	Frequently removed by other family members and not replaced.
Suitable for temporary use, easily removable.	Apt to dislodge upon rising, seat is not clamped to toilet.
Easy to install—just place on toilet seat.	Unstable.

Clamp-On

Advantages	Disadvantages
Sturdy.	Semipermanent.
Nonpadded seat; usually does not adhere to skin.	May be uncomfortable.
Padded seat is comfortable.	Padded seat apt to adhere to skin.
Easy to install—just fasten clamps to seat.	Difficult to clean under clamps without removing raised seat. Clothing may catch on elevated seat clamps when pulling garment up. Toilet seat always kept in raised position (can remove portable raised toilet seat and close toilet lid).
Usually includes inner guard to keep flow of urine from escaping.	Difficult for children to manage, especially young boys learning to stand to urinate.

TABLE 5. TYPES OF RAISED TOILET SEATS: ADVANTAGES AND DISADVANTAGES.

rocker knives, pizza cutters, one-handed cutting boards, nonspill mixing bowls, nonslip mats, and long-handled utensils.

Home health occupational therapy practitioners should carefully consider whether the items they offer will fulfill a real need for the individual's lifestyle. The person who rarely cooks and has historically preferred frozen dinners may not be interested in learning to use adapted utensils to prepare a meal, no matter how well these techniques make use of the patient's upper extremities.

C. Living Room Access and Use

Common living room barriers include carpeting and excess clutter. It is important to clear pathways and reduce clutter, particularly when patients are using mobility aids (e.g., a wheelchair, walker, or cane).

Chairs or couches often need to be raised in height so that patients can independently rise or transfer from their seat. Raising the height of the couch or chair by placing a second cushion (or 3-inch foam rubber cushion) on top of the first cushion can successfully increase the individuals ability to rise from their "soft" couch. Occasionally, a firm board can be placed underneath the chair cushion to provide more stability.

Inexpensive chair risers can be made by placing cement patio blocks under furniture legs for elevation. Four-inch square wooden blocks can also be

Problem	Possible Solutions
Slippery bathtub floor	Use rubber suction-grip tub mats.
Bathtub sliding glass doors prevent easy entry to tub	Remove doors from track. Substitute plastic curtain, hung with hooks and a spring tension bar.
Poor standing balance	Use bathtub bench or transfer tub bench.
Unable to clean perianal area	Use bathtub bench (often square-shaped) with keyhole opening, combined with use of long-handled sponge.
Limited funds for bathtub bench or bathtub seat	Use sturdy chair (e.g, molded plastic chair or metal kitchen chair with rubber crutch tips on feet; possibly covered with plastic trash bag, although watch safety due to slipperiness of plastic bag).
Bathtub bench too low	Utilize adjustable height bathtub bench legs.
Unstable sitting balance	Bathtub bench with a back. *Note: Bathtub bench backs may be contraindicated for large individuals due to their tendency to push a person forward.
Unable to enter bathtub standing up	Use bathtub bench with transfer board or transfer bench. Place one side in the tub and the other end placed outside tub; comes in padded or flat bench models.
Desire to sit in water, rather than on bathtub bench	Order bathtub hydraulic lift chair, with swivel seat, to aid transfers. Inflatable bathtub chairs are less costly, but be careful of patient's stability if recommending use.
Desire to control water flow	Recommend long-handled, hand-held shower hose with lightweight shower head. *Note: Control of water ideally located in shower head handle for individual to control, rather than on the wall, due to fluctuating water pressure. Also helps individual remain seated, rather than needing to lean forward to reach water controls.
Sporadic water temperature	Heat-sensitive safety valve installed in hot water line. *Note: Especially important for individuals with sensory deficits, those who live alone, or those who bathe unattended.
Family members want to use regular shower head	Use diverter valve, available in hardware stores; attaches hand-held shower hose to shower head, allowing dual use of regular shower head and hand-held shower hose.
Unable to stand or walk into shower or bathtub; unable to transfer onto bathtub bench	Recommend rolling shower chair; usually high-backed, waterproof chair with large back wheels; can be used independently by some clients (i.e., paraplegics); must have roll-in shower.
Unable to use bathtub	Utilize roll-in shower (no threshold); normally built by contractor according to American National Standards Institute specifications (ANSI, 1992).
Slippery bathroom scatter rugs	Remove scatter rugs to prevent slipping. If patient prefers rugs, stabilize them with carpet tape or substitute rugs with a rubber tub mat on the floor.
Unable to see mirror	Install mirror on wall at appropriate height. Install flexible mirror extenders or prop a mirror behind the faucets.

TABLE 6. BATHTUB BARRIERS AND ADAPTATIONS.

placed underneath each chair or couch leg. A 1-inch deep indentation chiseled in the top center of each block, carved to the size of the leg with the chair leg placed in the indentation, enhances safety and reduces the tendency for the chair leg to slide. Another way to make chair risers is to attach molding strips around the square block to help prevent the chair leg from falling off the block; particularly

helpful if an indentation cannot be carved. Overall, floor-to-seat height does not usually need to be higher than 21 to 22 inches (frequently a 4-inch rise) to enable a sit to stand transfer.

A platform frame, formed with 4 X 4 boards cut to the desired height and screwed or nailed into each corner of the frame, can be placed under a chair to increase chair height and facilitate an easi-

Problem	Solutions
Unable to reach sink from wheelchair	Remove sink doors. Remove cabinet threshold. Pad drain pipe with insulated rubber. Open sink doors and put feet on the inside shelf or threshold. Place overturned dishpan in sink and wash dishes on top of it to raise height of sink bottom. Use tilted mirror above sink to assist visual contact with dishes.
Unable to reach stove from wheelchair	Put tilted mirror above stove. Use long-handled utensils. Ideally, stove knobs should be located in front of stove. *Note: If stove knobs are in back, patient can use long-handled reacher or alternatives (i.e., potato masher). Discourage wearing long, flowing sleeves.
Unstable standing balance	May want to disconnect front burners to prevent patient from being burned. Use high stools with rubber feet. Movable high stools can be made by hammering nylon glides with spikes to bottom of stool legs, although make sure patient has good balance and cognitive awareness before recommending them.
Difficulty reaching into kitchen cabinets	Pull-out storage units. Turntables. Rearrange shelves so that frequently used items are on low shelves and special occasion items are on higher shelves. Reachers. *Note: Can make reacher bag for walker/wheelchair by sewing two pieces of material together to form long tube; tie tube to walker or wheelchair. Reacher with locking lever effective for those with limited grasp. Use regular kitchen or spaghetti tongs to reach items. Lower shelves.
Unable to transport items	Use two- or three-tiered wheeled cart; ideal with handles and feet with ball bearing casters that swivel 360°. Apron with large pockets. Wheelchair bags under or on back of wheelchair. Walker/crutch bags or baskets (beware of instability caused by too much weight in bags). Walker bags with pockets, ideally hung inside walker, to reduce chance of walker falling forward. Carry spillables (i.e., cup of coffee) in small dishpan. Place lids on all items that could spill, and on hot items.
Cannot reach/use countertop	Pull out medium height drawer and cover top with bread board, cookie sheet, or tray. *Note: Can cut large circle in center of bread board to stabilize mixing bowls.

TABLE 7. KITCHEN BARRIERS AND ADAPTATIONS.

Problems	Solutions
Door too narrow for wheelchair	Remove door. Remove door stops. Substitute a curtain for the door. Use alternate room. Replace door with an offset door hinge, available from hardware stores or Sammons catalog (Sammons, 1994).
Unable to maneuver over door threshold (sill)	Remove door threshold (sill). Place thin mat over door threshold to eliminate the threshold hump.
Unable to turn door knobs or faucets	Replace with levers. Provide knob turner.
Carpeting too think for easy maneuvering (i.e., shag)	Remove or replace carpeting; using indoor-outdoor carpeting is ideal for wheelchair and/or walking. Replace with tile floors.
Steps	Place handrails on both sides. *Note: If possible, extend railings beyond top and bottom step to allow individuals to continue holding on once they reach the top/bottom. Attach a door pull (i.e., U-shaped handle or sturdy knob) to door frame to give the individuals a sturdy handhold to grab. Install portable or permanent ramps (see following section on ramps). Use motorized stair glides—usually require at least a 22" stair width, although 28" stair width is recommended. Usually available for two levels of stairs. Consultation with a medical equipment dealer is highly recommended to assist in choosing and installing appropriate stair glide for the patient. Motorized porch lifts—require a firm foundation (cement pad), access to home entrance, and a safety gate to prevent falling off lift. Consultation with a medical equipment dealer is highly recommended to provide installation assistance and specific model and safety features needed for the patient.
Stair climbing	If patient cannot transport walker aids independently, a second walker, cane, or wheelchair may be needed on the second floor.
Floor surfaces	Eliminate throw rugs. Tape rug edges down with rug tape. Use larger rugs. Instruct patient to observe changes between floor coverings (i.e., rugs versus linoleum).
Electrical cords	Place around room perimeter. Tape to floor.
Furniture crowding	Discuss repositioning furniture with patient and family.
Doorbell ringing/access	Assess entrance way accessibility, ability to open/close door, ability to use door locks. Use flashing light system (or other visual identification) for hearing impaired.

TABLE 8. HOME ACCESS BARRIERS AND ADAPTATIONS.

er sit to stand transfer. The chair cannot slide off because of the restraint of the frame. Also, the ratio from chair seat to arm height has not been altered (such as when adding a second cushion to a chair).

Hydraulic easy-lift chairs (partially covered by Medicare on occasion) or portable chair lifts are available through DME dealers and can assist a patient rising from a chair or a couch. The patient needs to have a wide base of support and good balance in order to maneuver the chair lifts successfully.

D. Home Accessibility

The occupational therapy practitioner needs to be diplomatic and cost- conscious when recommending architectural changes to the patient's familiar environment (see Table 8).

Product/Part	Features
Wheelchair width	Many sizes available; standard adult wheelchair seat size is 18" wide. Usually, wheelchair seat width is 2" wider than patient's hips when sitting. Consultation with a DME dealer is recommended to help fit wheelchair if the occupational therapy practitioner has minimal experience in this area.
Wheelchair armrests	Full-length armrests allows more arm support; lap trays attach easily. Desk-length armrests allows wheelchair access under tables; do not provide patient with full arm support; can reverse desk arms to provide support during standing; does not easily hold a lap tray. Detachable armrests allows for lateral transfer; can reduce weight of wheelchair when removed. Nondetachable armrests are less expensive; cannot be lost; must transfer by standing up and moving forward rather than moving laterally.
Removable, swing-away footrests	Helps individual come close to a table or toilet, for example.
Wheelchair brakes	Always have patient (or caregiver, if patient unable) set brakes before transferring. Brake extenders are available for either side of the wheelchair, if patient is unable to reach brake lever or has limited upper extremity strength. Homemade brake extenders can be made from PVC pipe; cut and sanded, and placed over the brake.
Wheelchair tire rims	Smooth rims are standard. Knobby rims are available to facilitate grasp.
Wheelchair cushions	Numerous types and sizes of cushions are available. Skin integrity, weight of the patient, activity level, and cushion durability are all important factors to assess when choosing the appropriate wheelchair cushion. Solid seat cushions assist positioning and reduce body fatigue but can be uncomfortable for the frail, elderly individual. Consultation with a DME dealer regarding the numerous kinds of cushions available can help the practitioner make the appropriate recommendation.
Wheelchair backs	Majority of wheelchair backs rise to scapular level, although sports chair (common for para-plegics) may have lower back if individual using chair has good sitting balance. Sports chairs are usually lighter and used for increased speed and control. Higher raised-back chairs are often used for quadriplegic patients and those unable to independently support their backs.
Indoor and outdoor tires	Indoor tires: smooth, maneuver easily. Outdoor tires: knobby, stick to the surface well, may be slightly harder to push than indoor tires (due to increased traction), may track dirt into the home.
Hemi-chair	Wheelchair seat is approximately 2" to 3" lower than standard wheelchairs. Useful if patient uses legs to maneuver wheelchair. But, because wheelchair seat height is lower, it often prevents indi-vidual from using regular height table or counters from a sitting position.
Lightweight wheelchair	Significantly lighter than regular wheelchair. Easy for patient to maneuver since it is not as heavy. Easier for family members to lift. May not be as durable as standard weight wheelchair.

TABLE 9. COMMON FEATURES OF WHEELCHAIRS.

Ramps are occasionally recommended for use in the home health setting. A few of the major features of ramps are listed as follows:

- Can be portable (often 3 to 10 feet long).
- Available in a variety of surfaces and weights, from fiberglass to metal; heavier weights often used for power wheelchairs.
- Nonslip surface is ideal; can use nonslip strips available from most hardware stores. Also, paint can have sand added to make it a nonslip surface.
- Shallow walls needed on both sides of ramp to prevent individual from slipping off.

- Ramp height to stair height ratio, per ANSI, is a 1:12 ratio, meaning that for every 1 foot of elevation, 12 feet of ramp is needed for independent access (ANSI, 1992; AOTA, 1992). Assisted maneuverability is at least a 1:4 ratio, meaning that for every 1 foot of elevation, 4 feet of ramp is needed for an individual in a manual wheelchair to be pushed up a incline ramp. Contractors often give free estimates when quoting price and design for permanent ramp(s) and/or decks.
- A flat "deck" area is necessary immediately before the door, at the same height as the door bottom, to facilitate accessible entrance into the patient's home.

E. Wheelchairs

Patients often arrive home from a hospital or a rehabilitation center with a wheelchair. The home health occupational therapy practitioner needs to be familiar with the main features of a wheelchair in order to maximize both the individual's and the family's independence with this important therapeutic device (see Table 9 on p. 40). Therapists who are unfamiliar with wheelchairs, need to request assistance when making wheelchair recommendations.

VII. Occupational Therapy Equipment and Supplies

A car in good to excellent condition is the most important piece of equipment needed by home health occupational therapy practitioners. The car should have an adequate amount of storage space (preferably concealed) to facilitate easy access to evaluation and treatment supplies. Also, the car should be able to be driven in all types of weather and geographical conditions.

The home health occupational therapy practitioner is essentially a self-contained department. Practitioners carry all of their own testing equipment and supplies with them. Lightweight nylon or canvas gym bags with one or two zippered compartments can help therapists and assistants divide their supplies according to the problems being addressed (i.e., feeding equipment for evaluation and treatment in one compartment; equipment for bathing in another compartment; adapted equipment for grooming and dressing located in a third area). The amount and type of supplies will vary according to the number of patients the occupational therapy practitioner serves. Many occupational therapy practitioners will loan pieces of equipment to their patients for firsthand trials before recommending the purchase of these items. Some home health agencies do provide basic sup-

Items	Use
Pinch clothespins	Demonstrate/develop pinch strength. Wooden clothespins are often harder to pinch than plastic clothespins.
Wide elastic bands	Useful for strengthening fingers and finger abduction.
Sorting coins, nuts, bolts	Evaluate/treat finger dexterity and control.
Marbles, buttons, pins, paper clips	Improve unilateral and bilateral finger function.
Canned goods	A variety of sizes and weights can be used for strengthening and lifting exercises.
Rolling pins, sponges, washcloths	Upper extremity movements for shoulder, wrist, and grip strength.
Pulleys	Over the door hanger can be made with strong rope, PVC pipe, and a pulley from the hardware store. Place rope over the pulley and through the PVC pipe to make a handle; place over the door. Useful for active-assisted shoulder exercises.
Pouring from measuring cups and measuring spoons, turning doorknobs	Supination and pronation activities, wrist rotation.
Tableware, china, silverware	Use patient's own eating tools to evaluate and help maximize independent feeding skills.
Grooming items	Useful to evaluate and treat cognitive deficits. Work on manipulation skills and dexterity.

TABLE 10. COMMON OCCUPATIONAL THERAPY SUPPLIES FOUND IN THE PATIENT'S HOME.

plies, or have a loan closet, but this may not be the case in all situations.

Items found in the patient's own home can often be used very successfully by the home health occupational therapy practitioner. Patients are already familiar with items found in their home, there is no cost to either the patient or the practitioner, and the items are always present (see Table 10).

The types of equipment and supplies available to the home health occupational therapist and occupational therapy assistant are endless. Creativity is imperative in providing low cost yet appropriate therapeutic tools to facilitate a patient's successful functioning within the home and to ensure independence in self-care. Following are some examples of these low-cost tools:

- Blood pressure cuff
- Button hooks
- Cordless drill
- Dressing sticks
- Dynamometer
- Elastic shoelaces
- Fat pens and pencils
- Foam hair roller (disassembled and used to enlarge thin handles of items)
- Foam rubber
- Goniometer
- Inner lip plates
- Long-handled shoe horn
- Masking tape
- Reachers
- Rubber grip tape
- Stethoscope
- Tape measure
- Theraband® (or household elastic)
- Theraputty (or children's clay)
- Toolbox
- Velcro® (with and without sticky back)
- Vet Wrap® (for wrapping horse's legs): less expensive and used instead of Coban®

VIII. Conclusion

In today's health care arena, providing treatment in the home has become practical, cost-effective, and successful in helping to maintain an individual's functional independence. Evaluating and treating environmental safety needs, gross and fine motor coordination, daily living skills, and sensory, perceptual, and cognitive abilities are critical in the home environment. In addition, evaluating the need for splints, and facilitating the individual's involvement in appropriate leisure activities can help maximize the independence in their own environment. Assessing and alleviating architectural barriers throughout the home, and training the patient and family on appropriate use of DME can strengthen the success of the occupational therapy home program. Each occupational therapy practitioner needs to have their own specialized equipment and supplies in order to maximize the program. Family involvement, a patient's motivation, community support systems, and a

creative treatment plan that incorporates all of the above, will greatly influence the rehabilitation success of the patient with physical disabilities in the home. Occupational therapy practitioners working in home health have a unique opportunity to help patients and their families function well in their own home environment.

References

American National Standard Institute. (1992). *Accessible and usable buildings and facilities*. (Publication No. CABO/ANSI, A117.1-1992). Falls Church, VA: Council of American Building Materials.

American Occupational Therapy Association. (1992). *Resource Guide: Accessibility*. Rockville, MD: Author.

GAO study on Medicare's new prospective payment system flags potential hazards for older Americans. (1985m Spring). *Aging Reports*, p.1.

Health Care Financing Administration. (1986). *Home health agency manual* (Pub. 11). Washington, DC: U.S. Government Printing Office.

Hopkins, H.L., & Smith, H.D. (Eds.). (1993). *Willard and Spackman's occupational therapy* (8th ed.). Philadelphia: Lippincott.

Law, M. (1992). Evaluating activities of daily living: Directions for the future. *American Journal of Occupational Therapy, 47*, 233–237.

Pepper Commission. (1990). *U.S. Bipartisan Commission on Comprehensive Health Care, final report* (S. Prt. 101-114). Washington, DC: U.S. Government Printing Office.

Sammons catalog. (1994). Available from Sammons, P.O. Box 386, Western Springs, IL 60558-0386. 800-323-5547.

Chapter 6

Mental Health Services in the Home Health Setting: Special Considerations

by Judith A. Menosky, MS, OTR/L

I. Introduction

In recent years, the demand for mental health services for the homebound elderly population has increased. Thobaben (1989) and Harper (1989) identified major areas of need within the homebound population. Besides being mostly elderly, the majority receive Medicare coverage and cannot easily attend outpatient counseling. The homebound and their caretakers are susceptible to the stress associated with chronic illness, a loss of independence, a loss of significant others, and a sense of isolation. Over half of the homebound patients receiving mental health services had multiple medical illnesses such as cardiovascular disease, hypertension, diabetes, arthritis, cancer, stroke, and emphysema. Because of these varied needs, patients can often benefit from multiple services including nursing, personal care, social service, and allied health services.

The professionals meeting the demands of these patients are primarily mental health nurses who provide services for home health agencies (Richie & Lusky, 1987). Occupational therapy practitioners working in home health may encounter these patients as part of their caseload, or be part of a specialized multidisciplinary team that provides services to patients with mental health needs. Menosky (1990) states that homebound patients with psychiatric diagnoses often have difficulty with activities of daily living (ADL) due to the effects of mental illness and physical limitations. The occupational therapy practitioner can provide intervention in the areas of self-care, home management, environmental modifications, home safety, and the pursuit of avocational activities.

Occupational therapy is recognized by the Health Care Financing Administration (1989) as a reimbursable medicare service for homebound patients with a diagnosed psychiatric illness. Some specifics in the *Health Insurance Manual* (Health Care Financing Administration, 1989) that are evidence of this regulation include:

> Planning, implementing, and supervising of individualized therapeutic activity programs as part of an overall active treatment program for a patient with a diagnosed psychiatric illness. Example: use of sewing activities that require following a pattern to reduce confusion and restore reality orientation in a schizophrenic

patient. (Health Care Financing Administration, 1989, section 205.2)

Because homebound patients with psychiatric illnesses often have physical limitations as well, the skilled services included in the general description of occupational therapy can apply (Health Care Financing Administration, 1989). These services include activities to restore physical function, instruction to improve the level of ADL independence, and instruction in the use of adaptive equipment. This chapter will primarily address the patients who receive coverage under Medicare Part A because it is recognized that the majority of home health agencies bill for patient care under this part.

II. Service Delivery Models for Mental Health Services in Home Health

Two factors influencing the growth of mental health services in home health are earlier hospital discharges and the presence of psychiatric nurses in home health agencies. Occupational therapy practitioners have a specific role in the area of mental health services in this setting.

Occupational therapy practitioners often address the psychosocial needs of their patients regardless of diagnosis. For example, a patient recovering from a stroke may also experience depression due to a loss of functional abilities. If the symptoms are severe enough, a psychiatric nurse can be referred or share visits with the medical nurse. The occupational therapy practitioner can incorporate the patient's psychosocial needs into the treatment planning process and provide input to both nurses on the patient's progress.

A home health agency may take a more systematic approach by developing a psychiatric home health program. The Legacy Visiting Nurses Association in Portland, OR includes occupational therapy practitioners as part of a mental health team. Other team members include psychiatric nurses, medical social workers, physical therapists, speech-language pathologists, and home health aides. Gail Earle-Grimes (Earle-Grimes & Taegder, 1993), OTR/L and coordinator of the psychiatric program, feels that having a visible program enhances her agency's marketing efforts to referral sources including other agency staff, discharge planners, hospital social workers, and physicians. Earle-Grimes and a mental health nurse often make brief visits to physicians' offices to introduce their program. She states that, "Psychiatrists espe-

cially want to meet who is going to be working with their patients. It doesn't take that many doctors who support what you are doing to keep you busy" (Earle-Grimes and Taegder, 1993).

The mental health team also consults within the agency for patients with medical problems complicated by depression who are not progressing well with a medical or rehabilitative approach. This consultation provides for a holistic approach to each patient's care.

III. Homebound Status for Individuals With Psychiatric Diagnoses

In order to qualify for Medicare Part A coverage, a patient must be considered to be "homebound" according to Medicare guidelines. In the *Health Insurance Manual 11* (Health Care Financing Administration, 989), which describes these guidelines, a patient does not necessarily have to have severe physical limitations to qualify. However, they must need supervision to be considered safe outside the home, or must be refusing to leave home because of psychiatric symptoms. Some symptoms or problems that contribute to a patient's homebound status include:

- Diagnosis of dementia with impaired cognitive functioning
- Inappropriate or socially unacceptable behavior
- Disturbed thought processes or hallucinations
- Severe withdrawal or becoming reclusive
- Suicidal ideation or attempts
- Overwhelming anxiety or fearfulness

It is important that the primary service provider thoroughly describe and document the reason for a patient's homebound status. This is an individualized detailed description of why each particular patient cannot leave home without assistance or supervision and it justifies the need for home-based intervention (Harper, 1989).

IV. The Role of the Psychiatric Nurse

It is important that the occupational therapy practitioner understand the role of the mental health nurse in the home health agency because the nurse is an important team member, as well as a potential source of referrals. The mental health nurse is usually the primary service provider in cases where the patient has a diagnosed psychiatric illness and is under the care of a psychiatrist.

According to Medicare guidelines, the mental health nurse must have a nursing degree as well as additional experience in a psychiatric setting. The nurse is expected to work independently in the community to observe the patient's behavior and recommend any changes in the treatment plan to the physician. In addition, the psychiatric nurse's credentials need to be submitted to the intermediary for approval.

In home health, the mental health nurse has a multifaceted role. For the patient with a primary psychiatric diagnosis, the nurse serves as the primary service provider under the psychiatrist's plan of care. Since the patient usually sees a medical doctor as well, the nurse can function as a liaison between physicians, keeping them abreast of the patient's progress. The mental health nurse can also be requested by a medical nurse under a general physician's plan of care to evaluate a patient with an emotional or mental condition that is hindering recovery from an acute medical problem. A common example of this situation is the patient who develops depression in addition to having an exacerbation of a chronic medical condition. In this case, the mental health nurse can share visits with the medical nurse. In some instances, the mental health nurse can become the primary nurse as long as the medical needs are still addressed.

The need for mental health services in home health has been growing, and the role of the mental health nurse has been explored in recent literature (Richie and Lusky, 1987; Adams, 1989; Trimbath and Brestensky, 1990; Thobaben, 1989). The major tasks of the mental health nurse identified in the literature include a comprehensive evaluation of the patient in the context of the home and community environment; deciding whether the patient would benefit from a psychiatrist if one is not involved; educating the patient and caregivers about psychotropic medications; crisis intervention; and counseling and support for the patient and family.

V. Generating Occupational Therapy Referrals

As with obtaining any occupational therapy referral, the occupational therapy practitioner must educate referring agency staff and physicians about the nature and scope of occupational therapy services. A simple way to begin is by educating and communicating with the mental health nursing staff, if they are available in the agency. The mental health nurse may already have a working relationship with one or more psychiatrists and

can request an occupational therapy referral. A one-page sheet describing areas addressed by the occupational therapy practitioner, as well as good indications for a referral, can be provided for the nurse. An example of this type of information is found in Figure 11.

Main purpose:
To promote health and well-being by encouraging active participation and maximum independence in significant roles and daily activities including work, self-care, and leisure interests.

Occupational therapy can address the following functional deficits:
- Difficulty with home management and safety.
- Changes in cognitive, physical, or sensory function that reduce a person's level of independence in daily activities or jeopardizes personal safety in the home environment.
- Social withdrawal and difficulty adjusting to community living.
- Difficulty establishing a daily routine or setting short-term goals to promote recovery.
- Difficulty performing self-care activities (i.e., grooming, dressing, hygiene, transfers, functional ambulation).

Specific services
- Assess level of independence in self-care.
- Provide instruction to maximize the level of independence and safety in self-care.
- Recommend environmental adaptations or equipment to facilitate independence and safety in self-care and home management activities.
- Assess general cognitive function and assess the ability to participate in ADL.
- Explore and facilitate ways to participate in self-care and daily activities (i.e., home maintenance, social and community activities).
- Instruct caregivers in strategies to promote maximum participation, safety, and independence in daily activities for the patient.

FIGURE 1. OCCUPATIONAL THERAPY REFERRAL GUIDELINES FOR PATIENTS WITH A PSYCHIATRIC DIAGNOSIS.

Once an occupational therapy referral is received, it is essential for the occupational therapy practitioner to have ongoing communication with the mental health nurse and referring physician. This is a good opportunity to further educate other professionals about occupational therapy services as well as report on the patient's progress. An involved practitioner and a successful case example can go a long way towards promoting further referrals.

Home health occupational therapy practitioners who seek to include mental health referrals in their practice can find themselves sharing a case with many other disciplines, depending on the patient's needs. These include social services, physical therapy, speech-language pathology, and home health aides. Any of these disciplines can recommend an occupational therapy referral if approval is obtained by the physician. The recommendation should be communicated to the discipline that serves as the primary service provider.

VI. Functional Deficits Within the Homebound Psychiatric Population

The following list, while not necessarily comprehensive, identifies some of the major functional deficits that can be observed in the homebound population:

- *Failure to participate in daily activities and interests.*

  This can be a symptom of mental illness and can also be exacerbated by grieving issues associated with aging such as poor health, the death of family members or friends, and a decline in one's independence.

  Example: A woman with a history of depressive episodes suffered a recent CVA and has returned home after a month-long stay in a local hospital in a rehabilitation unit. Despite adequate performance of self-care and light homemaking skills during her stay at the hospital, she now feels too overwhelmed to resume her role as primary homemaker and assist in caring for her husband with chronic emphysema.

- *Social withdrawal.*

  When homebound, the sense of isolation is increased and previous social contacts may be lost. It can become more difficult to utilize transportation and community resources.

  Example: An 80-year-old retired male has just suffered an exacerbation of schizophrenic symptoms including auditory and visual hallucinations, and delusional thinking. After returning home from the hospital, despite experiencing a significant improvement in his psychiatric symptoms, he is staying in his bedroom all day. He refuses to say "hello" to neighbors, or go out to a local restaurant with family members once a week as he did previously.

- *Difficulty establishing a daily routine.*

  Independence in this area may be affected by physical, emotional, or cognitive deficits. The patient may feel too overwhelmed by problems to make constructive changes.

  Example: A 67-year-old female with major depression and recurrent psychosis has just returned home from a stay in a psychiatric inpatient unit for successful treatment of her symptoms. She also has diabetes and glaucoma in the early stages. Her husband works outside of the home, and she is alone for several hours on weekdays. She has had difficulty performing all hygiene and grooming tasks adequately. She is also having trouble getting organized in her role as primary homemaker. She does not utilize outside community resources, and family members (children and grandchildren) are usually not available to her except on weekends.

- *Deficits in self-care (grooming, bathing, dressing) due to emotional, sensory, cognitive, or physical deficits.*

  Example: A patient with a history of ministrokes has been experiencing increased difficulty with self-care due to paralysis and sensory loss on the right side, as well as deconditioning due to several hospitalizations in the past year. She is also experiencing a deepening depression since she had to give up her own home and move in with a family member.

- *Increased difficulty with home management and safety issues.*

  This includes performing housework, keeping track of finances, and cooking. There may be fall hazards in the home.

  Example: A patient with a history of schizophrenia returns home with family supervision after a recent hip fracture and surgery. The initial home evaluation reveals numerous fall hazards such as throw rugs in the bathroom and kitchen, a stairway with an inadequate railing, and poor lighting in the hallways and bedroom. The patient is resistive to making the recommended changes to improve safety because she likes the way things are and tends to deny the hazards.

- *Decreased physical strength and endurance.*

This is due to deconditioning after hospitalization or to chronic medical conditions.

Example: A 45-year-old woman with a recent exacerbation of multiple sclerosis is referred for home health services by her neurologist following a hospital stay. She has begun to experience more difficulty walking and considerable fatigue throughout the day. She experiences sensory loss that affects her coordination and ability to accomplish grooming tasks and meal preparation effectively. She is determined to keep up her present schedule and role as mother, wife, and homemaker, but often feels depressed and exhausted before noon each day.

- *Progressive sensory and cognitive impairment.*

This condition can involve vision, hearing, memory, and problem solving. It may be organic or due to medication side effects. It can also severely affect safety judgement and independence.

Example: An 80-year-old woman in the early stages of dementia has just returned home from the hospital following treatment for increasing confusion, agitation, dehydration, and anemia. She wants to return to living alone in her own home despite increasing problems with home management tasks including paying bills on time and cooking meals regularly. She is reluctant to accept community services such as Meals On Wheels and has had to rely increasingly on her daughter, who lives locally, for assistance with home management tasks.

VII. Occupational Therapy Frames of Reference Utilized With the Homebound Psychiatric Population

Three occupational therapy approaches are especially useful with the psychiatric population. The Model of Human Occupation (Kielhofner, 1985) takes a holistic view of a person's daily functioning and view of self. It is very applicable to use in the patient's home environment because this is the natural setting for the therapist and patient to explore values, roles, and habits. Together they are able to collaborate in setting functional goals that meet the patient's needs.

Claudia Allen's Theory of Cognitive Disabilities is also applicable as it provides a practical and measurable framework to assess cognitive deficits and their relation to daily activities. By using

Allen's cognitive levels as a basis for observing activities, as well as the Allen Cognitive Level Assessment (ACL) Tool, the practitioner can gain information that is useful in treatment planning as well as caregiver education (Allen, Earhart, & Blue, 1992).

The Rehabilitative Approach is also useful for patients with psychiatric diagnoses due to the frequency of physical and sensory deficits in the homebound population. It is still important to assess physical and sensory deficits, and environmental barriers. These patients can often benefit from programs addressing strengthening, energy conservation, and adaptive equipment needs.

VIII. Occupational Therapy Evaluation Guidelines

A specialized occupational therapy evaluation can be developed for the psychiatric patient, but a generic occupational therapy evaluation designed for home health practice will suffice as long as psychosocial issues are addressed. It is important to document how psychosocial dysfunction impairs the patient's ability to function to his or her potential. For example, documentation could read as follows: "Mrs. Jones is now experiencing severe depression and withdrawal affecting her ability to care for her personal needs, communicate with family members, or pursue daily home management activities and interests."

The major areas to be evaluated include the following:

- *Cognitive.*

Cognitive components include general alertness and orientation to surroundings, attention span, memory, judgement, and the ability to follow directions. The ACL test, a leather lacing task with graded levels of difficulty, can be utilized as an initial performance measure to determine the patient's cognitive level of function. This tool has some limitations, especially for patients with impairments in vision and fine motor coordination. A larger version is available to help reduce these limitations (Allen et al, 1992). The therapist in the home health setting can utilize the ACL test as part of the overall cognitive evaluation. It is recommended that the therapist compare the results from the test with observations of the patient's performance in selected ADL tasks, as well as consider a report from a reliable caregiver.

The Routine Task Inventory, as described by Allen (Allen et al, 1992) provides a useful framework for the therapist to use in gathering this information in the home health setting because observations can be made in the patient's natural setting and the primary caregiver is accessible to the therapist. The Routine Task Inventory is designed to be used to interview the patient and the caregiver, and observe task performance. The therapist can compare all these aspects to enhance the clinical picture of the patient's cognitive function.

* *Sensory and perceptual deficits.*

The therapist should identify deficits in vision, hearing, proprioception, and tactile areas. In a summary statement, it is important to indicate how the deficits impact daily functioning and independence.

* *Physical limitations: range of motion, strength, limitations in endurance, and activity tolerance.*

It is essential to identify the presence of complications such as deformities, pain, open wounds, and incontinence.

* *Medical history: Significant medical and psychiatric history.*

If the referral information is incomplete, ask the patient and caregiver about recent medical or psychosocial problems since the last hospitalization or within the past year. The therapist can confer with other service providers to confirm medical history.

* *Participation in major life roles and interests.*

This activity is determined through the interview process. Major roles include classifications such as homemaker, retiree, volunteer, or grandparent. Determining if any major losses or changes have occurred as a result of illness and what roles the patient desires to resume is essential. Interests can be assessed in much the same way. Some helpful tools include he Occupational Performance History Interview (Kielhofner, Henry, & Walens, 1989) and the Interest Checklist (Matsutsuyu, 1969).

* *Environmental contexts and safety issues.*

In home health, the therapist is in the ideal position to evaluate the patient's ability to function within his or her own environment. Some basic areas to assess are the patient's ability to maneuver safely, especially with an assistive device or wheelchair; the presence of safety hazards or fall risks; and the need for environmental modifications or adaptive equipment. The Kohlman Evaluation of Living Skills (Thomson, 1992) can be a useful tool for evaluating safety issues and judgment in more depth since it utilizes examples of safety hazards that are commonly found in the home setting.

* *Living situation.*

The occupational therapist (OTR) determines whether the patient lives alone or has a caregiver, has access to community services or outside supports, and the amount of supervision that seems appropriate. The OTR makes an initial determination of the patient's and caregiver's receptiveness to learn and follow a home program.

* *Recent psychosocial stressors.*

In collaboration with other service providers, the OTR can identify stressors that are contributing to the patient's decline in function. These factors may include family conflicts, financial problems, or inadequate housing. For example, a lack of financial resources can lead to poor nutritional habits and further deconditioning, all of which impacts the patient's ability to live at home safely. This information should be taken into consideration when developing the treatment plan.

IX. Occupational Therapy Approaches to Intervention

A. Psychosocial Approaches With Case Examples

The following psychosocial treatment approaches are meant only as a general guide. The practitioner is free to choose and implement various treatment approaches and activities with the patient. Approaches can be individualized to meet the patient's needs on a case-by-case basis. The main objective is to prevent hospitalization and improve the patient's independence and safety in all daily activities.

* *Participation in meaningful activities.*

The practitioner works with the patient and caregiver(s) to identify and facilitate the patient's involvement in meaningful tasks. The practitioner can suggest and demonstrate ways to modify the activity to match the patient's level of function. Adaptations, such as setting up the task appropriately and providing visual cues, can enhance the patient's participation in home activities.

* *Time management or balancing activities and roles.*

The occupational therapy practitioner works with the patient to analyze how the patient's daily routine is structured and how major life roles are balanced. This can be done through time management exercises (e.g., daily time log), and exercises designed to identify major life roles. Various time management and role identification exercises can be found in the book, *A Model of Human*

Occupation: Theory and Application (Kielhofner, 1985).

• *Goal setting.*

The therapist should involve the patient and caregiver as much as possible in setting short- and long-term goals. Setting short-term goals from session to session can be helpful in working with depressed patients. Goals can be reinforced in writing. The patient can also work on activities geared toward meeting goals in between occupational therapy sessions.

• *Coping strategies.*

The occupational therapy practitioner can work with the patient to identify methods to cope with daily stressors. Activities include relaxation techniques, paced breathing, problem-solving strategies, and role playing difficult situations. All of the coping techniques can be practiced within the context of a given activity (e.g., practicing some relaxation techniques with an anxious patient, and then planning a weekly schedule for meal planning and grocery shopping that breaks down into daily activities).

• *Socialization.*

The practitioner can work with the patient on deficit areas initially through home-based activities such as coping with home health visits, role playing, phone conversations, and inviting friends over to the home. These activities can progress toward the practitioner assisting the patient and caregiver in the identification of community activities and resources, and setting up a plan to begin implementing the chosen activities between therapy visits. It is important to elicit caregiver support yet encourage respite time for this person as well.

Case Examples

Case #1—A 67-year-old woman diagnosed with depression and major psychosis has just returned from a 3-week stay in an inpatient psychiatric unit. Her medical history includes diabetes and glaucoma. She does not leave her home except for medical psychiatric appointments and is unable to use transportation independently. She is a full-time homemaker and her husband works full-time outside of the home The occupational therapy evaluation revealed that the patient had the physical capacity to perform self-care tasks, but occasionally missed details due to visual deficits. Her main problem was an inability to organize her time and pursue her interests regularly or establish any type of community supports. She was strongly motivated to continue her homemaker role and to keep in touch with immediate family members in the area. However, she spent a lot of time alone, especially

on weekdays. She was often disorganized in her personal appearance and in completing homemaking tasks. Her cognitive impairment was mild with a score of 4.6 on the large ACL test.

Occupational therapy intervention focused on time management activities (using an activity configuration worksheet), further evaluation of home safety (especially meal preparation), improving participation with grooming tasks, identifying and pursuing leisure interests, and utilizing some community supports during the week. This patient displayed good potential to cook dinner daily and was able to compensate adequately for visual deficits after a few therapy visits. She exhibited significant deficits in personal hygiene and grooming, but over a 9-week period responded to short-term goal setting with grooming tasks and positive reinforcement for her efforts. She agreed to arrange for a beautician to visit her home once a week. She identified crocheting as an interest and was able to pursue it with a large crochet hook and a visiting companion to assist her in recalling patterns and providing support. Through support from her husband, the practitioner, and community volunteers, the patient was able to participate more effectively in daily activities. She was able to pursue a more balanced leisure and work schedule, and experience a sense of mastery and increased independence. She required ongoing community support to maintain this level of function and eventually attended a senior day-care program.

Case #2—An 80-year-old woman, who had been living alone, just returned home after a hospital stay. She was diagnosed with dementia in its early stages and put on medication to reduce agitation. The hospital treatment team recommended a supervised living situation, so the patient's daughter moved in while longer-term options were being considered. The patient was having more frequent periods of forgetfulness, especially in the late afternoon and evenings. She tended to deny her deficits and became angry when confronted with memory lapses. The occupational therapy evaluation revealed that the patient's cognitive deficits interfered significantly with home management tasks including money management, safe cooking activity, and handling novel or emergency situations. She scored a 4.2 on the ACL test.

This score indicated problem-solving deficits. She was able to accomplish familiar daily self-care tasks independently and use a shower with adaptive equipment. Occupational therapy intervention focused on educating the patient's daughter about the patient's level of function, need for supervision, and ways to promote active participation in activities at the patient's potential. For example, although the patient could not cook independently, she could participate in many food preparation tasks after all the materials were set up. Since the patient now required 24-hour supervision, the daughter agreed to hire a part-time caregiver. The caregiver provided the daughter respite, took care of household tasks, and provided stimulation for the patient by working with the therapist to plan and implement selected activities. With this structure, the patient displayed less agitation and increased independence in her ability to participate in her daily routine.

B. Rehabilitative Approaches With Case Examples

Because of the multiple needs often encountered with the homebound patient with mental illness, a basic rehabilitative approach can be utilized by the practitioner in conjunction with psychosocial approaches. Some common areas of intervention are as follows:

- *Skills training or retraining.*

This training includes self-care or home management skills that are identified in the treatment planning process. It is important for the practitioner to identify the patient's optimal level of function, choose appropriate activities, and modify the treatment plan as necessary.

- *Environmental modifications.*

These modifications can include removal of safety hazards including throw rugs and extra clutter, providing adequate lighting, marking steps, and rearranging furniture to accommodate an assistive device during ambulation. Most modifications can be done simply and inexpensively. If cognitive deficits are present in the patient, modifications such as visual cues and setting up self-care areas with needed equipment can greatly improve the patient's independence and safety.

- *Adaptive equipment needs.*

The practitioner should check bathroom equipment for compatibility with the patient's needs. The practitioner should also be aware that the patient's cognitive level influences the ability to use adaptive equipment effectively (Allen et al, 1992).

- *Graded activity programs.*

These programs can be beneficial for the recently hospitalized patient who has become deconditioned. They include general strengthening and range of motion (ROM) (e.g., chair exercises), instruction in paced breathing, energy conser-

vation, and body mechanics in the context of daily activities.

- *Caregiver instruction.*

This area is an important aspect of home health as the caregiver can have significant responsibility for implementing the home program. It is important to listen to the caregiver's concerns, provide support and education, and collaborate with him or her to devise and implement a realistic home program.

Case Examples

Case #1—A 68-year-old married male with a recent exacerbation of chronic obstructive pulmonary disease (COPD) has just returned home from the hospital and now has to use oxygen almost 24 hours a day. He has become increasingly depressed because of the seriousness of his condition and he has had to sharply curtail many previous activities including going out occasionally with friends, doing his own cooking, and walking his small dog. He now has increased support at home including a visiting nurse, a home health aide four times weekly to assist with bathing and transferring to tub seat safely, and Meals On Wheels. Physical and occupational therapy were referred to assist the patient in improving his level of daily functioning.

The occupational therapy evaluation revealed that the patient required moderate to maximum assistance in all self-care tasks except feeding, which was independent but with decreased appetite. Despite some ability to begin self-care tasks, the patient felt he did not know where to begin and passively allowed his wife and home health personnel to do all his self-care. Occupational therapy intervention focused on short-term goal setting to achieve specific tasks that the patient had as a priority such as using the shower again and getting dressed for the day. Instruction in energy conservation, self-pacing, and adaptive equipment were provided to the patient and his wife. The patient also agreed to participate in some mild upper extremity strengthening exercises.

Within 1 month, the patient was able to begin using the shower with a tub bench and wash his upper body with supervision only. He was able to dress himself with occasional minimal assist and began using adaptive equipment for footwear and slacks. He also felt encouraged to set new goals and continue working because, as he said, "I never thought I'd make it this far."

Case #2— An 82-year-old woman with a history of osteoporosis and depressive episodes was hospitalized when a large abdominal tumor was discovered that required an emergency colostomy. The patient was deconditioned upon returning home and was unable to resume many previous daily activities such as walking to various rooms, toileting, and getting dressed. She depended heavily on her husband for self-care and home management, and usually did not leave her bedroom. Despite education by the ostomy nurse, she was unable to begin caring for her colostomy. She also received home health aide services three times a week.

Occupational therapy was referred to assess ADL and equipment needs. The occupational therapy evaluation revealed that the patient had the potential to participate in self-care and functional transfers independently. The patient expressed anger at the sudden changes that had occurred due to her surgery and felt that she could not be seen by others this way. A referral was made for a mental health nurse to assist the patient in dealing with these feelings.

Occupational therapy intervention focused on short-term goal setting with self-care tasks, functional transfer tasks, and strategies to assist the patient in dealing with her fears of incontinence. When the patient realized that she would have to prepare for a doctor's office visit, she agreed to try wearing a protective pad and to get fully dressed. She also agreed to try having her commode frame placed over the toilet for daytime use. She was instructed in ways to begin participation in light homemaking at a modified level.

By the time she was discharged 2 months later, she was independent in dressing and grooming. She bathed with minimal assistance and walked regularly throughout her home with a quad cane. She began participating in her colostomy care with some assistance from her husband. She was able to express a positive sense of accomplishment with her progress.

X. Discharge Planning and Community Resources

The occupational therapy practitioner in the home health setting is free to work on preparing the patient for discharge without the same degree of pressure as in the hospital setting. If the patient is making progress in the 60-day period allotted by Medicare, the practitioner can plan accordingly. The practitioner can also plan for a shorter period of time if that is what the patient requires. In either case, the physician should be notified of the practitioner's plans.

The occupational therapy practitioner can work with the other treatment team members to explore and recommend a number of community services to assist the patient at home. These services can include those that may be funded by the county or state such as homemaking and personal care. These services begin after home health services have terminated including Meals On Wheels or an emergency response system such as Lifeline. The practitioner can also recommend follow-up care at an outpatient facility or mental health facility. In recommending these options, it is important to obtain a physician's order and to communicate with the other treatment team members since the patient will no longer be considered homebound under Medicare regulations.

Additional recommendations that can be made without a physician's approval include encouraging attendance at a local senior center that provides activities, or more planned outings with family and friends. For patients who remain truly homebound following home health services, some community resources may be able to come to the patient's home. These include beauticians, senior companions, and pastoral or church volunteers. The involvement of community resources can help ease the patient's and caregiver's transitions after home health services have terminated and provide a way for the patient to continue functioning at the highest level of independence.

XI. Documentation Considerations for Psychiatric Home Health

The documentation guidelines for occupational therapy practitioners working with psychiatric patients are essentially the same as those for general occupational therapy. The Health Care Financing Administration (HCFA), which determines the Medicare reimbursement guidelines, does not recognize specialty areas in occupational therapy. A major consideration for reimbursement includes the requirement that the patient needs skilled therapy services that can only be provided by an occupational therapy practitioner and that these services are considered reasonable and necessary by the intermediary for the patient's improvement in some aspect of daily functioning (Health Care Financing Administration, 1989). In addition, the patient must be considered to be homebound under Medicare guidelines for psychiatric patients (see discussion earlier in this chapter and in Chapter 8 on documentation). The guidelines can work to the practitioner's advantage when using a holistic approach to meet the multiple physical and psychosocial needs often found in the homebound population, regardless of the primary diagnosis.

Another important aspect for reimbursement is documenting the patient's needs and progress during treatment sessions. It is important for the practitioner to describe measurable changes and improvements in any aspect of daily functioning and the level of independence. For example, a note may read as follows: "On the initial occupational therapy visit this patient, recovering from depression and short-term memory loss, was neglecting personal hygiene tasks including washing her face and brushing her teeth on a regular basis. She required moderate assistance at least and prompting by her husband to complete these tasks. After 2 weeks of therapy, she performs these tasks independently, with only an initial reminder, after all the materials are set up within her visual range."

In 1990, an additional set of guidelines dealing with levels of cognitive function was added to the Medicare Part B guidelines (Health Care Financing Administration, 1990). Although these guidelines have not been added to Part A, occupational therapy practitioners will find them very useful as a guide for documenting the cognitive deficits present in their patients. They are also useful to determine the level of assistance needed and any improvements noted following therapy interventions. The guidelines break down the levels of cognitive assistance into the categories labeled as total, maximum, moderate, minimum, stand-by, and independent. Specific descriptions are provided for each category.

The guidelines can also be used for individuals with cognitive deficits that complicate recovery from either a medical or psychiatric condition. For individuals with a primary psychiatric diagnosis, the guidelines can be especially useful in documenting the need for further intervention. An example of documentation using these guidelines is provided in Figure 2 (p. 53) and the specific guideline descriptions are included in Chapter 8 on documentation.

Interventions provided by the practitioner that have an impact on the patient's safety in the home should also be documented. These can include the removal of safety hazards or instruction in the use of adaptive equipment recommended by the practitioner to enhance safety and ADL. It is also important for the practitioner to document any caregiver training that is necessary, especially for the patient who is cognitively impaired. It is acceptable to provide instruction over several sessions as long as it is not simply repetitive and progress is being made. For example, suppose the patient has demonstrated some impairments in safety judgement including forgetting to use a cane consistently and to turn off appliances in the kitchen. The caregiver is instructed of the need for increased supervision during meal preparation activities in ways to allow the patient to participate in this activity without having to be responsible for appliances.

XII. Conclusion

The provision of occupational therapy services in the home environment of individuals with psychiatric diagnoses is an exciting and rewarding area for occupational therapy practitioners to consider. The practitioner's training in functional evaluation, strategies to encourage independence in daily activities, and environmental modification is well-suited to the patient and caregiver training that is required in home health.

Recently, occupational therapy practitioners in the area of mental health began to reexplore the consumer's need for training in community living skills in community-based settings or hospital follow-up programs (Tomlinson, 1994; Baxley, 1994). The area of home health is a viable option, especially for those who are unable or not yet ready to participate in community programs following hospital discharge.

References

Adams, T. (1989). Growth of a specialty. *Nursing Times, 85*(40), 30–32.

Allen, C., Earhart, C., & Blue, T. (1992). *Occupational therapy treatment goals for the physically and cognitively disabled*. Rockville, MD: American Occupational Therapy Association.

Baxley, S. (1994). Options for community practice: The Springfield Hospital model. *Mental Health Special Interest Section Newsletter, 17*(1), 3–5.

Earle-Grimes, G., & Taegder, L. (1993, June). *Psychiatric home health in the 90's*. Speech presented at the 73rd Annual American Occupational Therapy Association Conference in Seattle, WA.

Harper, M.S. (1989). Providing mental health services in the homes of the elderly: A public policy perspective. *Caring, 8*(6), 5–9, 52–53.

Health Care Financing Administration. (1990). *Medicare intermediary manual, part 3, claims process* (DHHS Transmittal No. 1487, Section 3906.4). Washington, DC: U.S. Government Printing Office.

Health Care Financing Administration. (1989). *Health Insurance Manual, 11*, (Sections 204.1 and 205.2). Washington, DC: U.S. Government Printing Office.

Initial note:

Patient is a 69-year-old widowed female who lives alone in a senior citizen apartment. Supportive family members live locally. Admitting diagnosis is major depression. She was recently discharged from the hospital with follow-up from her psychiatrist, medical doctor, and home health services. Medical history includes diabetes, hypertension, osteoporosis, bilateral knee replacements, and a peptic ulcer. Home health services include a mental health nurse, home health aide, and an occupational therapist. Occupational therapy referral is for ADL evaluation, cognitive evaluation, and instructions in home safety.

Occupational therapy evaluation:

Cognitive function:

Patient is alert and oriented X 3. Scored 5.2 on the ACL. Demonstrates awareness of basic safety factors in the home, including the need to use her cane. Currently, the patient requires an increased level of community support including local family members and home health services to maintain her independence.

Psychosocial function:

Exhibits a decreased interest in self-care and previous social activities. Has difficulty establishing a daily routine. Expresses negative feelings toward self and others.

Physical and sensorimotor function:

No sensation or coordination deficits noted. Exhibits mild shoulder weakness (G–), and residual weakness in legs (feels unsteady without cane). There has been a sharp decline in activity level since her hospitalization as she has stopped doing conditioning exercises and does not leave her apartment for social activities.

ADL:

Demonstrates the ability to bathe, dress, and groom independently. However, interest in general appearance has declined. Home health aide supervises patient in the shower. The patient's ability to participate in meal preparation has declined, and she fears navigating in the kitchen.

Occupational therapy goals:

1. Return to all self-care tasks independently.
2. Return to light homemaking and meal preparation independently and safely.
3. Increase activity tolerance with homemaking tasks, and return to conditioning exercises independently.
4. Return to at least one leisure or social interest independently, or arrange community support as needed.

Plan:

Occupational therapy visits 1–2 times per week for 9 weeks for ADL retraining, home management tasks, exploration of avocational pursuits, and endurance activities.

Progress note:

Patient seen for a 50-minute session. Instructed to return to conditioning exercises established during a previous home health admission to prevent deconditioning. Patient able to begin program two times daily. Practiced and improved endurance for light homemaking activities in the kitchen for 10 minutes, and was able to get herself a light lunch. Patient stated that she experienced fatigue, but desires to do own cooking instead of getting Meals On Wheels. Given suggestions for easy-to- prepare meals for the following week. Began discussion of interests, and patient identified one activity within the building that she may want to pursue when she feels stronger. Currently, the patient requires minimal cognitive assistance to follow her home program including checks for the safety of kitchen activities and correction for occasional mistakes in conditioning program. Goals for next session: 1) Follow up with exercises twice daily 2) Prepare light lunch or dinner without assistance 3) Maneuver safely in kitchen during meal preparation tasks 4) Tolerate 15 minutes of activity before resting.

Discharge note:

Patient has demonstrated significant progress in ADL, home management, and pursuit of avocational interests. Can now initiate all self-care independently and no longer needs home health aide to use the shower. Prepares all meals independently and has improved general activity tolerance from 10 minutes to 30 minutes before needing to rest. Was initially very reluctant to pursue leisure and social interests but now attends a craft class in her building twice weekly. Plans to begin attending church with a family member. Still expresses sadness about her physical limitations and losing her husband. Plans to continue follow-up visits with her psychiatrist.

FIGURE 2. EXAMPLE OF HOME HEALTH DOCUMENTATION FOR PATIENT WITH A PRIMARY PSYCHIATRIC DIAGNOSIS.

Kielhofner, G. (Ed.). (1985). *A model of human occupation: Theory and application.* Baltimore: Williams and Wilkins.

Kielhofner, G., Henry, A., & Walens, D. (1989). *A user's guide to the occupational performance history interview.* Rockville, MD: American Occupational Therapy Association.

Matsutsuyu, J.S. (1969). The interest checklist. *American Journal of Occupational Therapy, 23,* 323.

Menosky, J. (1990). Occupational therapy services for the homebound psychiatric patient. *Journal of Home Health Practice, 2*(3), 57–67.

Richie, F., & Lusky, K. (1987). Psychiatric home health nursing: A new role in community mental health. *Community Mental Health Journal, 23*(3), 229–235.

Thobaben, M. (1989). Developing a psychiatric nursing home health service. *Caring, 8*(6), 10–14.

Thomson, L.K. (1992). *The Kohlman evaluation of living skills* (3rd ed.). Rockville, MD: American Occupational Therapy Association.

Tomlinson, J. (1994). The dimensions of occupational therapy in day programs. *Mental Health Special Interest Section Newsletter, 17*(1), 5–6.

Trimbath, M., & Brestensky, J. (1990). The role of the mental health nurse in home health care. *Journal of Home Health Care Practice, 2*(3), 1–8.

Chapter 7

Pediatric Services in the Home

by Rebecca Austill-Clausen,
MS, OTR, FAOTA

I. Introduction

There has been a tremendous increase of pediatric in-home services during the 1990s. The intent of these guidelines is to discuss the specific roles of the pediatric in-home occupational therapy practitioner. This chapter is not intended to be a treatise on pediatric services in general.

Effective pediatric home-based services require that the pediatric occupational therapy practitioner acknowledge and support family and parental involvement. Knowledge of the family's value system, socioeconomic culture, and sibling and parental relationships is essential to maximize pediatric in-home intervention (Hinojosa, Anderson, & Strauch, 1988).

Upon receipt of a referral for a child with special needs, home health occupational therapy practitioners should acknowledge whether or not they have the appropriate pediatric experience or the appropriate home health experience to adequately handle the situation. According to the American Occupational Therapy Association (AOTA) (1993b), it is the professional responsibility of the occupational therapy practitioner to consider themselves as an entry-level practitioner and ask for close supervision if they do not have appropriate pediatric training or adequate home health experience to provide in-home pediatric services.

II. Accessing In-Home Pediatric Services

A. Overview

There are a variety of ways that children can receive pediatric services in the home. Early intervention services are often provided in the home for children ages birth to 3 years. Pre-school-age children ages 3 to 5 years, and students ages 5 to 21 years can receive pediatric in-home services funded by the educational system, if deemed educationally appropriate. Children may require short-term in-home services due to an acute condition or accident that causes an inability to attend an on-site, center-based, or school system program (Hinojosa, Anderson, & Strauch, 1988). Children may receive privately funded in-home occupational therapy services either as a supplement to their educationally-based occupational therapy program or as a stand-alone service funded through their parent's insurance benefits. This care may also be funded by a managed care system such as a health maintenance organization (HMO) or a preferred provider organization (PPO).

Children with special needs do not need to be homebound in order to receive services at home.

Parents can request in-home treatment; a common occurrence for children receiving early intervention services. Frequently parents desire pediatric in-home therapy because of their inability to drive the child to a center due to a lack of transportation. There may be scheduling concerns and family issues that could be handled easier by a home-based treatment setting. Siblings may have nap schedules that conflict with scheduling at a center-based program. Parents may be unable to locate sitters to care for their siblings when bringing one of their children to a center for therapy (Gossens, 1993). Some children may become fatigued when travelling to center-based sites. Other children may be so medically fragile that they may not be able to attend a center- or school-based program. Therefore, in-home pediatric therapy would be essential for appropriate educational and therapeutic programming.

B. IDEA: Individuals With Disabilities Education Act

It is important for the in-home pediatric occupational therapy practitioner to understand the federal and state laws serving children that are ages birth to 21 years. When this document was written in 1994, the law serving children with delays was titled IDEA (Individuals With Disabilities Education Act) (IDEA, 1990).

IDEA is a federal law with state implementation. States can implement and interpret the law differently, but cannot be more restrictive than IDEA itself. For Part H of IDEA (covering services for children ages birth to 3 years), each state determines a lead agency to serve these children with special needs.

The lead agency, under IDEA Part B (serving children ages 3 to 21 years), is always the State Department of Education. However, states vary in their choice of a lead agency for programs serving children ages birth to 3 years. The lead agency may be the State Department of Education, the State Department of Health, or the State Department of Developmental Disabilities/Mental Health.

IDEA, Part B: Serving children 3 to 21 years old— In 1975, Public Law 94-142 entitled "The Education for all Handicapped Children Act" was passed. This law provided federal funds for "a free appropriate public education... in the least restrictive environment" to all children with disabilities within the age group of 5 to 21 years old (Education for All Handicapped Children Act, 1975). In 1990, this law was modified (PL 101-476) and called IDEA. It expanded the requirement for

educating disabled children to those ages 3 to 21 years. In this Act, occupational therapy is classified as a *related service,* and is required if the student's Individualized Education Plan (IEP) specifies the need for it (AOTA, 1993a).

Each student in special education has an IEP developed by a team of individuals working with the identified student, including the occupational therapy practitioner and always including the parents or guardians. The team agrees upon the appropriate type and amount of individualized services necessary to facilitate and maximize the student's educational program. Some students may have a need for in-home occupational therapy services. It is important that frequent communication occur between the educational program and the pediatric in-home occupational therapy practitioner. See Appendix F for a sample of an IEP format.

IDEA, Part H: Serving children birth to 3 years old—Since 1990, early intervention services for children ages birth to 3 years have been provided under IDEA, Part H. Initially in 1986, early intervention services were provided to children birth to 3 years, who were "developmentally delayed or at risk for developing delays" as classified under the Education of the Handicapped Act Amendments: PL 99-457 (1986). Often home-based programs are implemented as the most effective way to treat the child receiving early intervention services, in recognition of the home as the most natural setting, and being the least restrictive environment for young children. With the birth to 3-year-old population, occupational therapy is classified as a *primary service* in PL 99-457 (Schaaf & Gitlin, 1989).

Similar to the IEP in the educational system, early intervention services require that an Individualized Family Service Plan (IFSP) be written and that a case manager be identified to facilitate its implementation. Occupational therapy practitioners can serve as case managers in these situations (Case-Smith, 1990). Collaboration must occur between the professionals and the family members in order a child to receive the most benefit from their individualized program (Royeen, DeGangi & Poisson, 1992). See Appendix G for a sample of an IFSP format.

III. Referral Sources

Sources of pediatric in-home occupational therapy referrals include early intervention programs, neonatal intensive care units, acute care hospitals, outpatient clinics, home health agencies, occupational therapy practitioners, local pediatricians, day-care centers, infant-toddler programs, public health programs, parent-child centers, community pediatric programs, preschools, and day schools.

The provision of in-home pediatric services can be a fluid and shifting process. Children may receive acute pediatric services in the hospital, and be discharged to a pediatric in-home program. If the family has the resources, the desires, and the child is stable enough to attend a pediatric center-based program, the home program may be discontinued or supplemented by a pediatric center setting. If the child needs more center-based services due to increased socialization potential, increased availability of equipment, or greater access to team communication, the in-home program can be discontinued. It can be restarted at a later date if the team, in total collaboration with the family, feels that home-based therapy service could be beneficial at that time.

Some children may receive in-home pediatric service in the summer and then return to their school-based educational program in the fall. Other children, who are too ill to ever attend school, may also receive in-home services. Jane Case-Smith (1994) comments about the need for a "seamless system [that promotes]... best practice service delivery models that can meet the needs of all students in all settings" (p. 7).

Thus, practitioners providing in-home services need to coordinate and consult on a regular basis with the child's other team members. Effective team communication is especially important when therapy services are provided in a variety of settings and may use funding mechanisms different from IDEA, such as private insurance or Medicaid. Team consultation will also help provide the most constructive therapy programs for the child and their family.

IV. Evaluation and Treatment

A. Family-Centered Care Model

It is important to recognize that family members are the key components in all pediatric in-home services. The family makes the final decisions regarding the educational and therapeutic program provided to their child whether the services are provided in the home, in an educational facility, or in a combined home-based and center-based program.

The family-centered care model is essential to the effective delivery of pediatric services (Hanft, 1989a). It is important that in-home occupational therapy pediatric practitioners recognize the differ-

ences between the traditional medical model and the family-centered model. Pediatric in-home practitioners need to acquaint themselves with the consultative skills required to provide effective family-centered, collaborative treatment. McGonigel, Kaufman, and Johnson (1992) suggest that "professionals must be willing to go beyond the narrow boundaries of their disciplines or agencies and reach out to others who are also planning or providing services to these children and their families" (p. 2). Therapists need to realize that true family-centered care reflects the parents' (or primary caregivers') priorities and may not be identical to the priorities that the therapist would select (Hanft 1989b).

Schaaf and Gitlin (1989) quote numerous references in the literature that support the idea that a family-centered approach helps to maximize "positive behavioral changes in both the parent and the child... [and thus] decreases parental anxiety and stress" (p. 76). Hinojosa has conducted numerous studies about the impact that occupational therapy practitioners have on the lives of families with preschool-age children diagnosed with cerebral palsy. He recommends that practitioners may want to reduce their frequent use of child-centered home treatment programs. Instead, he asks practitioners to consider family-centered programs to help minimize the fragmentation that frequently occurs in families that have a child who is disabled (Anderson & Hinojosa, 1984; Hinojosa, 1990; Hinojosa & Anderson, 1991; Hinojosa, Anderson, & Ranum, 1988; Hinojosa, Anderson, & Strauch, 1988).

Case-Smith and Nastro (1993) studied the impact occupational therapy practitioners have on mothers and reached a similar conclusion. They suggest that mothers appreciate the "hands-on training, diagrams, pictures, and specific explanations... [and] written sheets with specific activities and recommendations for their children" (p. 816) when they are involved in home programs.

As in other home health settings, a pediatric home-based setting team of professionals includes the family, the child with special needs, occupational therapy practitioner, physical therapist, speech-language pathologist, social worker, psychologist, pediatrician, and teacher. The teacher often serves as the case manager in early intervention and preschool programs. The home medical equipment vendor may also be an integral component of the team, particularly for the medically fragile child. The team is often expanded for the older child and can include the above members plus the school principal, guidance counselor, adaptive physical education teacher, director of special education, related resource and learning room teachers, nurse, and district or school administrator.

B. Pediatric Diagnostic Categories

The following pediatric diagnoses are presented to acquaint the occupational therapy practitioner with those common in the home-based setting. Common pediatric diagnoses for infants receiving therapy in the home include prematurity; neuromuscular disease; congenital or genetic disorders; neurological insults occurring during, before or after the birth process; developmental syndromes associated with mental retardation; ventilator dependence; physical malformations and chromosomal abnormalities such as Down Syndrome; neuromuscular injuries associated with the delivery process such as brachial plexus; and children with parents having a history of substance abuse.

Other diagnoses common for pre-school- and school-age-children who may receive home-based services include those with spinal cord injuries, traumatic head injuries, terminal illnesses, orthopaedic disorders, mental retardation, developmental delays, muscular dystrophy, spina bifida, cerebral palsy, sensory integration disorders, learning disabilities, burns, emotional disturbances and behavioral problems, autism, juvenile rheumatoid arthritis, dyslexia, sensory disorders including visual impairments, and dyspraxia.

AOTA has a variety of one-page Health Professional Informational Sheets that may help acquaint the home health practitioner with pediatric services for specific diagnoses and situations (see Figure 1).

- Occupational Therapy for Children in School Settings
- Occupational Therapy for Individuals With Developmental Disabilities
- Occupational Therapy for Learning Disabilities
- Occupational Therapy in Early Intervention
- Occupational Therapy in Neonatal Intensive Care Units
- Occupational Therapy Services for Infants and Children

FIGURE 1. AOTA HEALTH PROFESSIONAL INFORMATIONAL SHEETS: PEDIATRICS.

C. Pediatric Evaluation in the Home

There are a variety of portable, standardized pediatric assessment tools available that can be used by the in-home occupational therapist (see Figure 2 on page 59). These assessment instruments can be used to supplement the in-home practitioner's observation of the child's natural home environment during the daily living activities, when playing with familiar objects or toys, and when interacting with the family. These activities all form a good basis for family-centered care.

D. Pediatric Treatment in the Home

Pediatric occupational therapy home-based treatment is a very effective way to facilitate maximal integration of the child's needs, the family's priorities, and the environment. The practitioner can observe the child and parent interacting in their own home environment and these observations can assist the practitioner in providing effective recommendations. In-home occupational therapy practitioners can evaluate the parent's ability to choose appropriate toys for their child, and advise the them accordingly about developmental levels. Practitioners can learn by direct observation about the family's priorities and needs, sibling relationships, and family motivation. Practitioners can observe the family's daily routine and provide applicable recommendations designed to facilitate their attempts to provide appropriate intervention strategies to the child within the context of the entire family unit (Schaaf & Mulrooney, 1989).

Occupational therapy practitioners in the home have the ideal opportunity to adapt treatment activities to the family schedule. They can also institute culturally appropriate practice. There are also many opportunities to develop trust and rapport with the family.

There can be a variety of types and frequency of in-home occupational therapy services provided to the child with special needs. Direct service can vary from one time per week or more to twice a month, or even one time a month, depending upon the needs of the child. In-home services can be primarily hands-on with family consultation, or primarily consultative, concentrating on family training. Small group sessions with other children are possible but sometimes difficult to arrange due to the logistics involved in getting two or more children together at the same home.

Treatment techniques in the home are family-centered. Helping family members understand the principles of specific positioning and handling

Bayley Scales of Infant Development (Bayley II) The Psychological Corporation 555 Academic Court San Antonio, TX 78204 (210) 299-1061	**Gesell Preschool Test for Evaluating Motor, Adaptive, Language,** & Personal-Social Behavior in Children 2 1/2 to 6 Programs for Education, Inc. PO Box 167 Rosemont, NJ 08556 (609) 397-2214
Beery-Buktenica Developmental Test of Visual Motor Integration (VMI) Modern Curriculum Press 13900 Prospect Road Cleveland, OH 44136 (216) 572-0690	**Hawaii Early Learning Profile (HELP)** Vort Corporation PO Box 60123 Palo Alto, CA 94306 (415) 322-8282
Bruininks-Oseretsky Test of Motor Proficiency American Guidance Service, Inc. 4201 Woodland Road Circle Pines, MN 55014 (612) 786-4343	**Miller Assessment for Preschoolers (MAP)** The Psychological Corporation 555 Academic Court San Antonio, TX 78204 (210) 299-1061
DeGangi-Berk Test of Sensory Integration Western Psychological Services 1203 Wilshire Boulevard Los Angeles, CA 90025 (310) 478-2061	**Peabody Developmental Motor Scales** Riverside Publishing 8420 West Bryn Mawr Avenue Chicago, IL 60631 (800) 767-8378 (800) 323-9540
Developmental Test of Visual Perception-2 (previously called the Marianne Frostig Developmental Test of Visual Perception) Pro Ed 8700 Shoal Creek Boulevard Austin, TX 78757-6897 (512) 451-3246	**Quick Neurological Screening Test** Academic Therapy Publications 20 Commercial Boulevard Novato, CA 94949 (415) 883-3314
Early Intervention Developmental Profile The University of Michigan Press PO Box 1104 Ann Arbor, MI 48106 (313) 764-4392	

FIGURE 2. COMMON PEDIATRIC ASSESSMENT TOOLS USEFUL FOR THE IN-HOME OCCUPATIONAL THERAPY PRACTITIONER.

techniques, oral stimulation strategies, sensory processing, neuromotor concepts, developmental play, cognition, and appropriate adaptive techniques for daily living skills are frequent goals of the in-home occupational therapy practitioner. There are often more consultation services, rather than direct services provided, when treating in the home. Because the practitioner and the family work together to identify problems and strategies, collaboration is essential no matter what kind of therapy intervention is used.

E. Conflict Resolution

IDEA provides for a specified legal grievance process to occur if either the child or family are dissatisfied with their educational or early intervention program (IDEA, 1990). Yet, if the IFSP and the IEP are developed in a collaborative manner responsive to the family's needs, most conflicts can be avoided. Every program providing pediatric services should have an internal conflict resolution process that can be implemented immediately upon realization of a family concern. If the internal conflict resolution process is unsuccessful, a trained mediator should be made available to help the family and program practitioners to resolve any concerns. A formal administrative grievance procedure can also be utilized at any point if the family or agency desires (McGonigel et al, 1992).

This formal due process hearing requires a trained, impartial compliance officer to resolve the conflicts. Parents, or the aggrieved party, can appeal any decision by asking for a review by the lead state educational agency, or the local, state and finally the federal courts. Occupational therapy practitioners may be called to testify as to the need, frequency, and type of occupational therapy services recommended and provided (AOTA, 1989). If true collaboration between the family and the pediatric program has occurred, this formal conflict resolution process should be unnecessary.

V. Therapy Equipment and Supplies for the In-Home Pediatric Practitioner

Equipment, toys, and play activities brought to the home by the in-home pediatric occupational therapy practitioner must be portable, lightweight, durable, and easily carried from the practitioner's car into the child's home. It is the practitioner's responsibility to clean and disinfect any toys or equipment that they supply and that have come in contact with the child's body fluids (e.g., drooling).

One of the benefits of providing care in the home is the ability to utilize the child's own toys. Modeling appropriate developmental play activities with the toys can serve as an excellent teaching example for parents and other family members. Often, because children are familiar with their own toys, the practitioner can use their interest to help stimulate appropriate developmental progress.

Figure 1 includes suggestions for portable pediatric therapy equipment along with a variety of supplies appropriate for the in-home pediatric occupational therapy practitioner. Often pediatric practitioners bring a canvas or nylon bag, filled with toys appropriate to the situation, into the child's home for demonstration, treatment, and training purposes.

Occasionally, the pediatric in-home practitioner is involved in selecting appropriate positional equipment, seating systems, or wheelchairs for children. A well-trained pediatric durable medical equipment (DME) dealer, or rehabilitation technology supplier, can be a great asset to the practitioner. The dealer can be asked to bring sample products to the home to be evaluated by the entire family and custom fitted for the child. The DME dealer should be familiar with Medicaid and other commercial carrier billing procedures. It is helpful to ask the vendor to submit the appropriate paperwork for reimbursement. Also, it is advised to ask the dealer which items are covered by Medicaid, private commercial carriers, or other relevant funding sources prior to making a decision to purchase the equipment.

VI. Documentation Considerations

Documentation requirements for the pediatric occupational therapy home-based practitioner

---

Equipment

- T-Stool
- Bubbles
- Scooterboard
- Brushes
- Vestibular board (can be made from plywood and two wooden rockers underneath)
- Textured cloths
- Spinning saucer (can use metal or plastic disc sold commercially for sledding)
- Developmental toys from local toy stores
- Small trampoline
- Target games
- Cardboard boxes and packing cases for tunnels
- Small cuff weights
- Cardboard tubes covered with cloth
- Different sized balls
- Heavy cardboard containers covered with carpeting
- Puzzles
- Carpet squares
- Coloring books
- Different size plastic buckets for a small sand table
- Bean bags
- Use family's sink for water table (Byrne, 1976)
- Different textured rug samples
- Homemade chairs: Triangle chair, Cylinder chair, Roller chair, Corner chair (Finnie, 1978)
- Rice, beans, lentils for tactile activities
- Gymnastic balls
- Vibrators
- Laptop computer or other portable video games
- Foam balls
- Electronic toys
- Switch dogs

FIGURE 1. EXAMPLES OF PEDIATRIC THERAPY EQUIPMENT FOR THE IN-HOME OCCUPATIONAL THERAPY PRACTITIONER.

often depends upon where the service is being provided, and who is the funding source. For example, if home-based services are being provided through an early intervention center (for children ages birth to 3 years), the occupational therapy practitioner will be required to participate in the IFSP process that includes specific documentation requirements. The written IFSP is reviewed periodically, at least every 6 months, and includes an annual evaluation by all involved disciplines.

The IFSP form is completed during a meeting of team members including the parents. Agency policy and family priorities determine how many of the team members are present for the actual meeting. If an occupational therapy practitioner is unable to attend, a written occupational therapy report is helpful to assist the IFSP team in writing goals. McGonigel, Kaufman, and Johnson (1992) suggest that "the IFSP—the written product itself—is possibly the least important aspect of the entire IFSP process. Far more important are the interaction, collaboration, and partnerships between families and professionals that are necessary to develop and implement the IFSP" (p.1).

If in-home occupational therapy services are provided to school-aged children ages 3 to 21 years, an IEP is developed as the working document. The occupational therapy practitioner is expected to collaborate with the team members, write annual goals and short-term objectives, anticipate service duration, and evaluate criteria for the occupational therapy component of the IEP.

Occupational therapy goals provided in the IEP for children between the ages of 3 to 21 years must be educationally relevant. Thus, the practitioner needs to justify the occupational therapy program in educational terms. For example, a goal to increase a child's fine motor skills would be rephrased in educational terms to say that fine motor skills are necessary to help children complete their school-work more efficiently and effectively.

Documentation needs will vary greatly, depending upon the funding source and agency requirements. Medicaid and insurance companies may be looking for documentation to reflect the "medical" model of treatment , rather than the educational model (Case-Smith, 1994).

Children may have a medical, adaptive, or developmental need that does not affect their education but that affects their function at home or in the community. In this case, service provided by a private practitioner or community-based organization, or reimbursed by an insurance company may not reflect the child's educational need. However, goals and objectives would still need to be developed in accordance with a child's IEP or IFSP to obtain maximum benefit and coordination among all service providers. All occupational therapy practitioners providing pediatric services in the home are strongly encouraged to consult with the appropriate funding source and their respective agencies regarding the required documentation.

VII. Discharge Planning

Occupational therapists and occupational therapy assistants can discharge a child from occupational therapy before other team members do if the team feels that discharge is merited in this area of therapy. Discharging a child from in-home occupational therapy services to a center-based intervention program or school system requires clear communication and collaboration with the other team members and especially with the child's family. Acquainting the family to community resources, funding mechanisms, outpatient services, advocacy programs, equipment vendors, service directories, local pediatric programs, and other professional contacts is a necessary component of the discharge process.

It is recommended that a final discharge summary be written that itemizes the initial and final date of service, frequency, duration and overview of the in-home occupational therapy service, goals achieved, and occupational therapy recommendations. Providing the family with a copy of the written discharge summary is an excellent way to make sure that they are aware of the in-home occupational therapy practitioner's recommendations. With the family's permission, a copy should also be sent to the receiving agency. Families should be given the opportunity to respond to any concerns that they may have regarding the discharge planning process or the occupational therapy discharge report. Communication and collaboration with the family is an essential ingredient of home-based family-centered care.

VIII. Reimbursement

Reimbursement for in-home pediatric services is varied and can include funding from federal programs such as Medicaid, and Maternal and Child Health Programs. State and community agencies such as the Department of Mental Health or Mental Retardation/Developmental Disabilities may also fund services. Local agencies such as the Lions Club and the Chamber of Commerce are also possible payers of pediatric services and equipment.

IDEA, Part H, which covers children ages birth to 3 years, allots funds to supplement, not supplant, existing funding sources. IDEA, Part B, covering children ages 3 to 21 years, reports that the State Department of Education is responsible for all programs for children with disabilities within the state, but that other funding sources may also be tapped such as Medicaid and private insurance companies (IDEA, 1990).

Funding pediatric in-home programs through commercial insurance carriers and managed care plans varies according to each family's individual policy or plan. It is highly recommended that a written authorization be received from the insurance carrier or managed care provider prior to implementing in-home pediatric service. Authorizations should include an official written clarification of the insurance company or managed care plan requirements for home-based service, rates, expected service duration, and documentation needs.

IX. Conclusion

The provision of in-home pediatric services is an exciting and challenging environment for occupational therapy practitioners. The majority of children receiving this type of therapy are ages birth to 3 years. Although, home-based services are also provided to children ages 3 to 21 years with special needs. Utilizing a family-centered collaborative model as the basis for all treatment and training recommendations is one of the most effective ways to serve the child with special needs in the home.

References

American Occupational Therapy Association. (1993a). *The importance of occupational therapy services provided under IDEA: The need for advocacy.* Rockville, MD: Author.

American Occupational Therapy Association. (1993b). Occupational therapy roles. *American Journal of Occupational Therapy, 47*(12), 1087–1098.

American Occupational Therapy Association. (1989). Occupational therapy issues in due process hearings. In the American Occupational Therapy Association *Guidelines for occupational therapy services in school systems.* (2nd ed.). (pp. 10–1 to 10–9). Rockville, MD: Author.

Anderson, J. & Hinojosa, J. (1984). Parents and therapists in a professional partnership. *American Journal of Occupational Therapy, 38,* 452–461.

Byrne, J.M. (1976). *Early intervention program resource guide: Selected readings from programs for young disabled children in Pennsylvania.* Harrisburg, PA: Pennsylvania Department of Public Welfare/Office of Mental Retardation.

Case-Smith, J. (1994, July). *Testimony of the American Occupational Therapy Association on the Reauthorization of the Individuals with Disabilities Education Act.* Presented before the House Education and Labor Committee Subcommittee on Select Education and Civil Rights, Washington, DC.

Case-Smith, J. (1990). Case management in early intervention. *American Occupational Therapy Association Developmental Disabilities Special Interest Section Newsletter, 13* (4), 5–8.

Case-Smith, J. & Nastro, M. (1993). The effect of occupational therapy intervention on mothers of children with cerebral palsy. *American Journal of Occupational Therapy, 47,* 811–817.

Education for All Handicapped Children Act, PL 94-142, (1975).

Education of Handicapped Act Amendments, PL 99-457, 20 U.S.C. Sections 1400–1485 (1986).

Finnie, N. (1978). *Handling the young cerebral palsied child at home.* New York: E.P. Dutton.

Gossens, M. E. (1993). The child in the home. In May, B.J. (Ed.), *Home health and rehabilitation: Concepts of care* (pp. 330–332). Philadelphia: F.A. Davis Company.

Hanft, B.E. (1989a). *Family-centered care: An early intervention resource manual.* Rockville, MD: American Occupational Therapy Association.

Hanft, B.E. (1989b). Nationally speaking—Early intervention: Issues in specialization. *American Journal of Occupational Therapy, 43,* 431–434.

Hinojosa, J. (1990). How mothers of preschool children with cerebral palsy perceive occupational and physical therapists and their influence on family life. *Occupational Therapy Journal of Research, 10,* 144–161.

Hinojosa, J. & Anderson, J. (1991). Mothers' perceptions of home treatment programs for their preschool children with cerebral palsy. *American Journal of Occupational Therapy, 45,* 273–279.

Hinojosa, J., Anderson, J. & Ranum, G.W. (1988). Relationships between therapists and parents of preschool children with cerebral palsy: A survey. *Occupational Therapy Journal of Research, 8,* 285–297.

Hinojosa, J., Anderson, J., & Strauch, C. (1988). Pediatric occupational therapy in the home. *American Journal of Occupational Therapy, 46,* 17–22.

Individuals with Disabilities Education Act, PL 101-476, 20 U.S.C., Sections 1400–1485 (1990).

McGonigel, M., Kaufmann, R., & Johnson, B. (1992). *Guidelines and recommended practices for the individualized family service plan* (2nd ed.). Bethesda, MD: Association for the Care of Children's Health.

Royeen, C.B., DeGangi, G., & Poisson, S. (1992). Development of the individualized family service plan anchor guide. *Infants and Young Children, 5* (2), 57–64.

Schaaf, R.C. & Gitlin, L.N. (1989). Early intervention: New directions for occupational therapists. *OT in Health Care, 6* (2/3), 75–89.

Schaaf, R.C. & Mulrooney, L. (1989). Occupational therapy in early intervention: A family-centered approach. *American Journal of Occupational Therapy, 43,* 745–754.

Chapter 8

Special Considerations Affecting Documentation in Home Health

by Judith A. Menosky, MS, OTR/L,

with contributions from Velma Reichenbach, MS, OTR/L, and Mary Jane Youngstrom, MS, OTR

I. Introduction

The demands on occupational therapy practitioners for documentation of service continues to challenge those providing therapy in the home health setting. In order to ensure reimbursement, the documentation must adhere to the rules established by service providers, government agencies, and accreditation organizations while also proving the necessity and uniqueness of occupational therapy as a skilled health care service (Reichenbach, 1992).

Although occupational therapy practitioners may be focusing on the actual provision of services, it is documentation that will demonstrate the importance and value of occupational therapy services to anyone who reviews the case at a later date. This includes Medicare intermediaries or reviewers from within the home health agency.

Therefore, it is essential that all documentation be clear and complete.

An article by Allen, Foto, Moon-Sperling, and Wilson (1989) states that "improper documentation can result in a claim being denied or returned to the provider for additional information thus jeopardizing the patient's access to further treatment" (p.783). Similarly, Gillard and Kern (1991) suggested that "every plan of treatment (claim) submitted to an intermediary represents an opportunity to educate a third-party payer. Every plan of treatment written and submitted to a third-party agency is an act of patient advocacy. The quality of our documentation is a measure of our professional credibility. Clear and accurate documentation reflects sound clinical reasoning."

II. Important Considerations for Medicare Part A Documentation

A. Homebound Status

The patient must be considered homebound. This means that leaving home could be medically contraindicated, or requires considerable effort and assistance in the form of close supervision or the need for special equipment and transportation services. The patient's homebound status should be documented upon evaluation and periodically thereafter, as long as the case is open. A diagnosis alone is usually not enough; functional limitations must be described in some detail.

The following are examples of patients who qualify as homebound:
- The patient requires the use of a walker and the close supervision of a caregiver at all times.
- Due to severe shortness of breath and limited endurance, the patient can only ambulate 20 ft before needing rest.
- Due to the patient's periods of confusion and loss of contact with reality, a caregiver must accompany the patient to all appointments.
- The patient needs 24-hour supervision due to impairments in judgment and a history of frequent falls.

B. Addressing the Physician's Orders

If the initial occupational therapy orders require an evaluation of activities of daily living (ADL) skills and adaptive equipment needs, then the occupational therapy evaluation should clearly address these areas with function and outcome as the frame of reference. If the practitioner feels there is a need for further intervention, the physi-

cian's approval must be obtained according to the home health agency's policy. This process can include a phone call to the physician's office and generally requires the physician's signature on the occupational therapy evaluation and treatment plan, as well as on the Home Health Certification and Plan of Treatment—HCFA Form 485 (see Appendix H).

During the course of treatment, if orders need to be added or changed, then a form provided by the agency for this purpose can be used. Some examples of changed or updated orders include:
- Requested approval to progress to hand-strengthening exercises.
- Requested approval to reduce visit frequency to once weekly, due to the patient and caregiver's progress in following the home program.

C. Occupational Therapy as a Skilled Service

The patient must have a clearly identified need for skilled occupational therapy services. These services are defined as "skilled" when they can only be performed by a qualified occupational therapist or occupational therapy assistant. This includes instruction to the caregiver in a home program that requires the supervision of the occupational therapist to establish, monitor, and change it as necessary.

The following are examples of occupational services:
- The patient and caregiver were instructed in safe positioning techniques and methods to reduce edema in the affected upper extremity.
- The patient and caregiver were instructed in the use of a button hook to facilitate independence in dressing.
- The patient, who lives alone, was instructed in energy conservation techniques and practiced them while preparing lunch during the occupational therapy session.
- The patient and caregiver were warned about cooking hazards that a patient with these particular cognitive deficits may not notice.

D. Intermittent Visit Pattern

Therapy should be provided on an intermittent basis to meet the patient's rehabilitation needs. Therapy services are not usually required daily, as in the acute care or rehabilitation hospital, but the practitioner can establish a regular weekly visit pattern to create a home program and instruct the patient and caregiver.

The following are examples of visit patterns:
- Occupational therapy 2 to 3 times per week for 9 weeks for ADL training.
- Occupational therapy 2 to 3 times per week for 4 weeks, then 1 to 2 times per week for 4 weeks for upper extremity muscle reeducation program, ADL training, and adaptive equipment needs.

The visit pattern can occur in a range, such as 1 to 2 times per week or 2 to 3 times per week, depending on the intensity of visits required to implement the treatment plan. For example, three visits a week may be required for the first 2 weeks; then the visit frequency can be reduced to 2 times per week after the practitioner feels that the patient and caregiver are following up with the treatment plan and making progress towards goals.

A frequency range can also allow for visit cancellations due to medical appointments without having to obtain an order change from the physician. However, some agencies may require that the physician always be notified if a visit is canceled. It is important that occupational therapy practitioners become familiar with the agency's policies regarding establishing visit frequencies and adhere to these policies.

E. Reasonable and Necessary

The skilled therapy services must be considered reasonable and necessary based on the occupational therapy practitioner's evaluation. This can mean that the practitioner expects the patient to demonstrate functional improvement within a reasonable period of time, or that therapy services are necessary to establish a safe and effective maintenance program.

The following are examples of progress during therapy sessions:
- The patient has improved from moderate to minimal assistance in bed to chair transfers.
- The patient can now participate in meal preparation using the walker with only occasional cues for safety.

It is also important to document the need for continued therapy sessions for either rehabilitation or maintenance programs. The following are examples of this type of documentation:
- Patient and caregiver exhibited difficulty following up with self-grooming techniques due to patient's continued neglect of the left side and limited attention span. Continued instruction was provided to the caregiver in breaking down the task for the patient and reducing the length of practice sessions.

- Patient requires 1 to 2 follow-up sessions to ensure that maintenance range of motion program is performed safely and consistently according to the guidelines established.
- Psychosocial example: The patient and caregiver exhibit a conflict after participating in a light housekeeping routine recommended by the occupational therapy practitioner due to the patient's lack of awareness of mental difficulties and the caregiver's response by blaming the patient for neglecting the task. Continued instruction was provided to assist the patient in sweeping the floor within his abilities and to demonstrate some verbal cuing techniques the caregiver could utilize to assist the patient in completing the task.

F. Establishing a Maintenance Program

A maintenance program can be established by an occupational therapist and then monitored, with help, by an occupational therapy assistant. According to the guidelines in section 205.2 of the Health Care Financing Administration's *Health Insurance Manual* for Medicare-certified home health agencies (1989), a therapist can establish and monitor a maintenance program when it is documented that the skills of the occupational therapy practitioner are required to manage and periodically reevaluate the effectiveness of the program and also to insure that the patient and caregiver implement the program safely. Most agencies require that the occupational therapy practitioner limit the maintenance program to a specified period of time because visits performed for maintenance have a greater risk of being denied. Occupational therapy practitioners are encouraged to be aware of and follow the agency's guidelines when establishing and monitoring such a program.

The following is an example of a patient in need of a maintenance program:

A patient must use a resting hand splint for night wear as part of the home program. The patient and caregiver demonstrate good follow-up of the program during an intensive visit pattern of 2 to 3 times per week. The practitioner may gradually reduce the visit pattern, and because of the identified dangers of skin breakdown or edema during splint wearing periods, may choose to monitor the program at a reduced frequency of 1 time per week for 2 weeks, then 1 time every 2 weeks for 1 month to ensure safe follow-up of the home program over a longer period of time.

G. Avoiding Duplication of Services

When working on similar areas of function, practitioners in different disciplines should collaborate and avoid documentation that would look like a duplication of services.

The following are examples of methods to avoid this duplication:

- Both the occupational therapy and physical therapy practitioners can work on transfer skills and can avoid duplication by emphasizing different functional aspects. The physical therapist can emphasize lower extremity strengthening, balance, and posture. The occupational therapy practitioner can concentrate on safety judgement and recommend the appropriate type of adaptive equipment to facilitate the transfer.
- The occupational therapy practitioner and speech-language pathologist can both address cognitive skills of the patient who is recovering from a stroke. The speech-language pathologist can engage the patient in cognitive exercises that involve verbal processing of memory and problem-solving skills. The occupational therapy practitioner can work with the patient on a daily living task to address the same skills. The documentation must reflect the different approaches used to address functional skills.

H. Words or Phrases to Use or Avoid

The following examples are of words or phrases that can be problematic, but do not have to be if they are more clearly stated.

- Avoid the word "maintain." It indicates that the patient has reached a plateau. Medicare does not pay for maintenance except under special circumstances as noted earlier. A statement such as "Treatment was provided to maintain function" should be avoided as well. If there has been a plateau, and new strategies to reverse the plateau have not been successful in a short time, then discharge would be advised. However, a practitioner may provide skilled services by setting up a maintenance program.
- The phrase "making slow progress" should be avoided. The phrase "steady progress" may more accurately describe the client's progress toward functional goals.
- Do not say: "Patient is not progressing." Instead, give the reason why progress has been inhibited. Describe the practitioner's plan such as "patient placed on hold," or

say that "changes in goals and treatment were made as a result of the problem."

- Verbs such as "review," "reinforce," or "reinstruct" should be used carefully because they make it appear that the service is repetitious, or that the patient has not been compliant or was not able to comprehend.
- Avoid using statements such as "generalized weakness" instead of stating specific functional limitations such as shortness of breath after climbing a specific number of steps, poor balance, dizzy, or unsteady gait. Generalized weakness is usually thought of in conjunction with an illness where intervention is not required to increase strength or where age is the cause of the weakness. Instead, make a specific statement about a functional limitation and the need for further intervention.
- Avoid generalized statements that are not objective or measurable such as "healing well," "responding well," and "good endurance." Be more specific about the changes. Statements should be behavioral and measurable.
- Indicate that the patient is in need of skilled services. Insurance company intermediaries may look at training in self-dressing or passive range of motion as nonskilled. It may be perceived as something that could be administered by untrained personnel or a family member unless there is something in the documentation that shows the uniqueness of your work with the patient. For example, self-ranging may be performed in such a way as to be a part of neurodevelopmental treatment. Dressing can incorporate specific neurodevelopmental or muscle reeducation techniques that also address the improvement of strength and range of motion of a weakened upper extremity. Backward chaining may be necessary in working with another type of patient due to cognitive deficits. Similarly, dressing training may address the perceptual dysfunction by increasing awareness of body parts when unilateral neglect is present (Reichenbach, 1992).

I. Documenting the Need for Cognitive Assistance

Medicare recognizes the role of occupational therapy in treating the cognitive deficits associated with psychiatric and physical disabilities. The regulations issued by the Health Care Financing Administration (HCFA) in 1990 clearly define the levels of assistance that can be used to describe the patient's current functional status. Each level defined (total, maximum, moderate, minimum, stand-by, and independent) includes a description of the individual's physical needs for assistance as well as the degree of cognitive assistance required (e.g., one-to-one demonstration, intermittent verbal cuing, or help in correcting mistakes (HCFA, 1990). The inclusion of these cognitive parameters in Medicare's understanding of function more clearly defines occupational therapy's role in the treatment of individuals with psychiatric problems and those individuals with physical diagnoses complicated by cognitive deficits. Table 1 outlines the types and levels of physical and cognitive assistance that can be used to document change (see Table 1).

J. Writing Functional Goals

To satisfy the requirements of third-party payers and intermediaries, occupational therapy goals must be written in functional terms in a manner that is clear and measurable. Goals must address specific functional activities such as self-care or home management tasks. Progress towards goals must be documented in terms of measurable and observable improvements related to some aspect of daily functioning. At the same time, they should reflect a need for further skilled intervention (Mahoney & Kannenberg, 1992).

Goals should address what the patient or caregiver will accomplish, not what the occupational therapy practitioner will do. For example, phrases like "Provide instruction to the family on bathroom safety and equipment," or "Instruct in one-handed dressing techniques" would be a part of the practitioner's plan. If a statement can be preceded with "patient will..." or "caregiver will...,"

Assistance Level	Physical Assistance	Cognitive Assistance
Total	100% assistance by one or more persons to perform all physical activities.	External stimuli are required to elicit automatic actions such as swallowing.
Maximum	75% assistance by one person to physically perform any part of a functional activity.	Cognitive assistance such as 1:1 demonstration or sensory input is needed to perform gross motor actions in response to direction.
Moderate	50% assistance by one person to perform physical activities.	Constant cognitive assistance such as intermittent 1:1 demonstrations or physical or verbal cuing are needed to sustain and complete simple, repetitive tasks safely.
Minimum	25% assistance by one person for physical activities. Set up or help needed to initiate or sustain performance.	Periodic cognitive assistance is needed to correct repeated mistakes, check for safety compliance, or solve problems presented by unexpected hazards.
Stand-by	Supervision by one person to perform new procedure adapted by practitioner for safe and effective performance. Patient does not use safety precautions and demonstrates errors in performance.	
Independent	No physical assistance.	No cognitive assistance.

TABLE 1. LEVELS OF ASSISTANCE.

Table adapted from *Medicare Intermediary Manual, Part 3, Claims Process* (DHHS Transmittal No. 1487, Section 3906.4) by the Health Care Financing Administration, 1990, Washington, DC: U.S. Government Printing Office.

then it is an appropriate goal. Examples of functional goals include:

- The patient will prepare light meals safely and independently in the home.
- The patient will dress independently except for minimal assistance with footwear.
- The patient will pursue two leisure interests on a regular basis with close supervision of the caregiver.
- The patient's daughter will implement a home activity program independently with the patient. The program will consist of the patient's active participation in one leisure interest and one household task of interest.

An effective method to establish a treatment plan is to write long- and short-term goals that are defined in functional terms. Goals that are functional and measurable provide guidance to the occupational therapist and occupational therapy assistant in establishing a clear treatment plan and documenting progress from session to session (Mahoney et al, 1992; Denton, 1987). In home health, the long-term goals can encompass the 60-day certification period, while short-term goals may cover a few sessions to several weeks within that certification period. Short-term goals must be related to a long-term goal and are usually updated and changed more often. Short-term goals may also address the functional components of the skills identified in the long-term goal such as improving upper extremity range of motion and strength to accomplish a grooming task with less assistance. Some examples of the goal setting and treatment planning process are as follows:

Example 1: In this example, the patient lives at home alone and is receiving Meals On Wheels following hospitalization. She would like to eventually discontinue Meals On Wheels and prepare her own meals.

Long-term goal: The patient will prepare light meals safely and independently at home.

Short-term goals:

- Within 2 weeks, the patient will independently follow an upper extremity strengthening program designed to increase endurance for homemaking tasks.

- In the next week, the patient will demonstrate safe maneuvering techniques in her kitchen while using a walker.

- Within the next month, the patient will prepare one light meal daily.

Treatment plan:

- The occupational therapy practitioner will provide instruction in the upper extremity strengthening program.

- The practitioner will instruct the patient in safe maneuvering techniques with a walker, providing adaptations in her kitchen as needed.

- The practitioner will instruct the patient in the use of energy conservation techniques during light meal preparation.

Example 2: In this example, a patient with severe cognitive deficits is not expected to become independent, but hopes to participate actively in selected activities with the caregiver's assistance. The goals are addressed towards the caregiver's implementation of the treatment plan.

Long-term goal: The patient's daughter will implement a home activity program independently with the patient consisting of the patient's active participation in one leisure interest and one household task of interest.

Short-term goals:

- Within the next 2 weeks, the patient and daughter will choose a leisure interest with the occupational therapy practitioner's assistance.

- Within the next 2 weeks, the patient and daughter will choose a homemaking task with the occupational therapy practitioner's assistance.

- Within the next 4 weeks, the patient and daughter will explore various ways to adapt one chosen task to match the patient's residual cognitive function with the guidance of the occupational therapy practitioner.

Treatment plan:

- The occupational therapy practitioner will educate the patient's daughter about the level of the patient's cognitive impairment as well as her residual abilities and how this affects her task performance in daily functional activities.

- The occupational therapy practitioner will instruct the patient's daughter in methods and adaptations to use with the selected activity that will promote the patient's active participation.

In summary, both long- and short-term goals must be clear, measurable, and understandable to the intermediary. Clear goal setting will facilitate the practitioner's ability to establish an effective treatment plan and provide a clear indicator of functional outcomes.

III. Types of Documentation Required for Medicare Part A Coverage

A. Documentation for the Occupational Therapist

1. Occupational Therapy Evaluation

This evaluation is usually completed on a form provided by the home health agency and covers the various performance areas and components commonly addressed by occupational therapists. These include ADL such as feeding, grooming, bathing, toileting, dressing, bed mobility, and functional transfers. Instrumental ADL include homemaking, money management, and home safety awareness. Performance components of ADL skills include cognition, safety judgements, perception, sensory processing, upper extremity sensation, coordination, range of motion, and strength. Important environmental factors to consider in the evaluation include accessibility of the home, adaptive equipment that would benefit the patient, assistive devices being used, and the presence of a caregiver or community services. These items are often addressed in a checklist format where the occupational therapy practitioner identifies areas of impairment and the amount of assistance the patient requires for each daily living skill. As part of the evaluation, the practitioner usually includes a clinical summary written in narrative form, which summarizes the major areas of need and provides justification for continued occupational therapy services, if needed.

Finally, the occupational therapy goals and plans for intervention must be identified. Following is an example of a narrative note with initial evaluation findings:

> The patient is a 78-year-old female with an onset of a left CVA and right hemiplegia on March 9, 1994. Past medical history includes hypertension and insulin dependent diabetes. The patient was seen for an occupational therapy home evaluation on March 20, 1994 following a 2-week hospital stay. The patient lives on the first floor of a two-story home with her elderly husband. She is now receiving home health aide services 3 times weekly for personal care and receives Meals On Wheels. Prior to the CVA, the patient was independent in all self-care and light homemaking tasks.

The occupational therapy evaluation reveals deficits in short-term memory, problem solving, and sequencing with previously familiar self-care tasks such as bathing and dressing. A right visual field cut is present. The right upper extremity exhibits impairment with fair minus strength, abnormal flexor tone, and limitations in active range of motion to 0–90 for shoulder flexion and abduction. Fine motor coordination is significantly impaired. Sensation is moderately impaired in light touch, proprioception, and stereognosis.

In self-care tasks, the patient requires moderate assistance in all areas except feeding, which requires supervision and cuing. Transfers require moderate assistance to all surfaces to stand and pivot.

Occupational therapy goals and treatment plan:

Within the initial certification period of 8 weeks, the patient will accomplish the following:

- Improve bathing and dressing skills to minimal assistance.

- Improve functional transfers to and from bed, wheelchair, and commode to minimal assistance.

- Participate in one to two light homemaking tasks of interest with set up and minimal assistance of the caregiver.

Within the next 4 weeks, the patient will:

- Demonstrate an increased awareness of her right side during self-care tasks by attending to the right side with minimal cuing.

- Consistently follow one- to two-step instructions with familiar self-care and light homemaking tasks.

- Participate in a muscle reeducation program for the right upper extremity designed to facilitate participation in self-care tasks with minimal assistance of the caregiver.

Occupational therapy plan:

Occupational therapy visits 2 to 3 times per week for 8 weeks for muscle reeducation program, cognitive and perceptual retraining, and ADL training. The rehabilitation potential appears fair to good for accomplishing the previously stated goals within this time period. The patient is expected to remain at home with 24-hour supervision provided by the caregiver(s). The patient's progress and the need for further occupational therapy intervention will be reassessed within 8 weeks.

2. Discharge Summary

This summary should include the dates of occupational therapy services, the patient's progress and present level of function, the reason for discharge, and follow-up plans.

> Example: This patient was seen for occupational therapy services from March 20, 1994 to June 30, 1994. In this time, the patient has made significant progress in self-care tasks including dressing, which has improved from moderate assistance to independent for the upper body and minimal assistance for the lower body.
>
> Bathing has improved from moderate to minimal assistance to wash the back and left arm, and the patient is able to transfer to a tub seat with minimal assistance. Transfers have improved from moderate to minimal assistance to stand and pivot to the chair or bed. The patient began to participate in some light food preparation tasks while sitting, and stands at the sink for 5 minutes before fatigue.
>
> Some residual weakness and impaired coordination remains in the right upper extremity, but a gross grasp is present, and the patient can grasp and stabilize objects from 2"–4" in diameter.
>
> Patient is being discharged because occupational therapy goals have been met, and she is functioning at her maximum potential at home. The follow-up plan is to be evaluated for outpatient therapy after her next doctor's visit in 2 weeks.

3. Initial Note

This note is a statement that the occupational therapy evaluation has been initiated or completed. It can be the first entry of the care plan where further occupational therapy interventions will be documented.

> Example: The occupational therapy evaluation was completed on March 9, 1994. The patient exhibits deficits in cognitive and perceptual function, upper extremity function, and ADL. Approval for further occupational therapy intervention will be sought from the referring physician. See the occupational therapy evaluation for more detail.

4. Progress Note

A progress note is usually written for each visit. A checklist or flow sheet format can be used to identify the major areas of intervention, followed by a narrative summary at least once a week. However, requirements may vary between agencies. It is important to state specific improvements in function, continued deficits, the need for further teaching, and updated goals as necessary.

> Example: The patient was seen 3 times this week for ADL training, cognitive and perceptual retraining, and muscle reeducation program for the right upper extremity. The patient exhibits progress in following one-step instruction during dressing tasks. She was able to don a pullover top with minimal assistance and cuing by the practitioner to begin on the affected side. The husband was instructed to work on this task with his wife for the next week. The patient has also begun to perform self-range of motion exercises two times daily for the past week and has achieved 120° passive range in the right shoulder. She requires verbal cuing and initial demonstration to complete each exercise. Updated goals:
>
> • In the next week, the patient will don her pullover top with verbal cuing only.
>
> • The patient will perform three range of motion exercises for the right upper extremity with verbal cuing only.

5. Communication Notes

The requirements for these types of notes can vary between agencies. However, Medicare intermediaries do require some type of documentation that demonstrates communication between disciplines, when applicable. Agency service providers may be providing excellent care and coordination of the patient's case, but only documentation can demonstrate that this is occurring.

Documenting communication is a valuable practice for the practitioner to acquire for several reasons. It provides tangible evidence of coordination between disciplines and can demonstrate collaborative treatment planning, especially after each discipline has completed an initial evaluation. It can also be helpful to document when the initial contact with the patient and caregiver was made and the approximate date set for the initial visit. Finally, documentation can explain the reason for a missed visit or a change in visit frequency. These notes need not be lengthy, but should provide a clear explanation with the essential details.

Here are some examples of communication notes:

• The patient was seen for the initial occupational therapy evaluation on (provide date). Continued treatment will be provided in the areas of self-care skills, cognitive and perceptual retraining, and instruction in the use of adaptive equipment. Treatment goals discussed with physical therapy, speech, and restorative nurse.

- The patient was contacted at home via a phone call on May 2, 1994. The initial occupational therapy visit was scheduled for May 4, 1994.

- The patient was seen for only one occupational therapy visit this week because of a doctor's appointment that conflicted with the visit schedule.

- The patient was unable to be seen for an occupational therapy visit as scheduled this week due to severe weather conditions and the patient feeling ill. The physician's office was notified of the canceled session. The primary nurse was also notified.

6. Supervisory Note

When documenting supervision provided for the occupational therapy assistant, it is important that the occupational therapist be aware of regulations set up by state licensure boards, which can vary from state to state. Supervision can include communication of the results of the occupational therapy evaluation and treatment plan to the occupational therapy assistant, case management, determining program termination, providing instruction and assistance as needed, and periodically observing the occupational therapy assistant. Supervision can occur through one or several different opportunities: face-to-face communication, telephone contact, the review of written notes, or group conferences (The Pennsylvania State Board of Occupational Therapy Education and Licensure, 1992). The supervisor needs to maintain a supervisory plan and document each supervisory contact with the occupational therapy assistant. It is recommended that occupational therapy practitioners use several approaches during the supervisory period.

Example of an occupational therapy supervisory note:

- The occupational therapy evaluation was completed on June 21, 1994. The evaluation results, goals, and treatment plan were communicated to the occupational therapy assistant, who will implement the treatment plan with a visit pattern of 2 to 3 times per week for 8 weeks. The occupational therapist will provide an on-site supervisory visit with the occupational therapy assistant by the sixth treatment visit.

B. Documentation for the Medicare Plan of Treatment

Medicare has devised three required forms for all disciplines that provide home health services with the information used to justify reimburse-

ment for services rendered. All of the forms are published by the Health Care Financing Administration (HCFA) under the Department of Health and Human Services. The forms are summarized as follows:

1. 485 Home Health Certification and Plan of Treatment

This form includes identification information of the beneficiary (patient) and the provider of services (home health agency). The initial orders for each discipline are written including treatments and frequency, and duration of services. The goals and rehabilitation potential are identified. It is sent to the physician for a signature. The occupational therapist provides information for occupational therapy orders and treatment, functional limitations, activities permitted, and rehabilitation goals and potential (see Appendix H for example of the 485 form).

2. 486 Medical Update and Patient Information

This form is completed at the end of the first month after home health services are initiated and serves as a monthly summary before the end of the certification period, which is 60 days. Each discipline is required to provide a summary of clinical findings and include any updated orders. The homebound status of the beneficiary must also be described and updated. The occupational therapy practitioner provides input in each of these areas. The signature of the nurse or practitioner completing the form is required (see Appendix H for an example of the 486 form).

3. 60-Day Summary or Recertification

In home health, the initial certification period to receive Medicare coverage is 60 days. In that time period, the Initial Home Health Certification and Plan of Treatment (485 form) and the Medical Update and Patient Information (486 form) are sent to HCFA. If any home health discipline identifies a need for services beyond the 60-day certification period, then recertification for the next 60 days must be requested of the physician for a new certification plan (485 form). For the occupational therapist, this involves a reevaluation of the patient's status and any updated orders. Then the same process would continue for the next 60 days.

C. Documentation for the Certified Occupational Therapy Assistant (COTA)

The COTA can write any note that is not exclusively required for the occupational therapist. These notes include case conference notes, progress notes, monthly summaries, and discharge summaries. It is recommended that all notes written by the occupational therapy assistant be cosigned by the occupational therapist. See the examples in the following sections.

1. Initial Visit Conference Note

After the occupational therapist has completed the initial evaluation, a conference will be conducted with the COTA via a phone call or in person. The occupational therapist will share the evaluation findings and expected functional outcomes with the COTA. The COTA will document the conference in the following way:

> The occupational therapist completed the initial evaluation on 4/15/94. The evaluation findings, expected functional outcomes, and goals were discussed via a phone conversation. The treatment plan established will include occupational therapy visits two times weekly for 8 weeks by the COTA to work towards treatment goals.

2. Documentation of Supervisory Visit

The COTA should participate in a joint supervisory visit with the occupational therapist. The required frequency of supervisory visits can vary according to state licensure laws or home health agency policies. The occupational therapy practitioner needs to be aware of all applicable regulations. During the supervisory visit, the occupational therapist observes the treatment session and provides input to the progress report.

The occupational therapy practitioner will collaborate with the assistant to establish updated goals and treatment plans. The COTA writes a note for the session. The following is an example of such a note:

> (Provide date) The occupational therapist and occupational therapy assistant completed a supervisory joint visit in the patient's home. Treatment goals and plans were updated in the following manner: 1) Improve dressing skills to independent with the use of adaptive equipment 2) Improve functional transfers to independent 3) Begin preparing a light meal at least once daily utilizing energy conservation principles.
>
> Plan: Continue progressive ADL training, transfer training, and instruction in energy conservation techniques. Occupational therapy visits to continue 2 to 3 times weekly for 5 weeks, then the need for further services will be reassessed.

A joint supervisory visit may be an ideal scenario. Licensure laws and agency policies vary from state to state. The important thing to remember is that supervisory contact between the occupational therapist and COTA must occur at regular intervals while a case is open, and be clearly documented.

3. Interdisciplinary Communication Note

When the COTA assumes the primary responsibility for implementing a treatment plan in a given case, he or she may also assume responsibility for documenting any interdisciplinary communication that takes place. All conferences should be documented whether they took place via phone or in person. Medicare requires documented evidence of interdisciplinary communication. Each discipline should sign his or her individual report or a summary report prepared for the conference. It can be helpful for each team member to receive a written copy of the report. The various disciplines should have ongoing communication to provide continuity of care. The following is an example of an interdisciplinary communication note:

> The occupational therapy assistant and physical therapist discussed the patient's progress toward treatment goals and coordinated the scheduling of visits. Plans to coordinate treatment approaches to maximize the patient's attainment of rehabilitation goals were shared.

Table 2 summarizes the essential notes that are required for proper documentation in the home health setting (see Table 2). The entries are categorized according to the occupation therapy practitioner who is responsible for the particular note.

Type of Note	OTR's Responsibility	COTA's Responsibility
Occupational Therapy Evaluation	■	
Initial Note	■	
Progress Note	■	■
Discharge Summary	■	■
Supervisory Note	■	■
Interdisciplinary Communication	■	■
485 Initial Orders	■	
486 Monthly Summary	■	■
60-Day Summary Recertification	■	■

TABLE 2. SUMMARY OF DOCUMENTATION REQUIRED IN HOME HEALTH.

IV. Conclusion

It is important to remember that documentation is the primary evidence to reimbursement sources and outside reviewers that competent occupational therapy services were provided. It should be clear, concise, and adhere to Medicare requirements, state licensure laws, and the home health agency's policy. Occupational therapy practitioners should be willing to continuously improve their skills in this area. Effective documentation can demonstrate that home health care is a valuable and cost-effective service for the patients served.

References

Allen, C., Foto, M., Moon-Sperling, T., & Wilson, D. (1989). A medical review approach to Medicare outpatient documentation. *American Journal of Occupational Therapy, 43,* 793–800.

Denton, P.L. (1987). *Psychiatric occupational therapy: A workbook of practical skills.* Boston: Little Brown.

Gillard, M., & Kern, S. (1991, June). *Application of AOTA uniform terminology to practice: Guidelines for documentation.* Paper presented at the American Occupational Therapy Association Conference, Cincinnati, OH.

Health Care Financing Administration. (1990). *Medicare intermediary manual, part 3, claims process* (DHHS Transmittal No. 1487, section 3906.4). Washington, DC: U.S. Government Printing Office.

Health Care Financing Administration. (1989). Health Insurance Manual 11, (Section 204.1). Washington, DC: U.S. Government Printing Office.

Mahoney, P. & Kannenberg, K. (1992). Writing functional goals. In J.D. Aquaviva (Ed.), *Effective documentation for occupational therapy.* Rockville, MD: American Occupational Therapy Association.

The Pennsylvania State Board of Occupational Therapy Education and Licensure. (1992). Title 49, Professional and vocational standards (Chapter 42). *Pennsylvania Bulletin, 22*(18), 2337.

Reichenbach, V. (1992). Special considerations II: Home health. In J. Acquaviva (Ed.), *Effective documentation for occupational therapy.* Rockville, MD: American Occupational Therapy Association.

Chapter 9

Quality Management in Home Health

by Caroline Higgins,
OTR/L, CPHQ

with contributions from
Michael J. Steinhauer,
OTR, MPH, FAOTA,

I. Introduction

Just as the role of occupational therapy in home health provides for unique and specialized practice components, there is also a unique role of and need for quality management in the home health arena. The use of quality management techniques in a home health environment will vary widely, depending upon the size and complexity of the organization. A separate home care agency that affiliates with a hospital may have its quality management program organized through the hospital quality management department, or it may have its own designated individual or department. In many free standing agencies, the quality management functions may be incorporated into one or several existing positions. Taking into account these variations, there are similarities in all settings relative to the role of the home health occupational therapy practitioner in quality management.

Why do quality management anyway? Why all this focus on proving that quality care occurred? We know we are performing well and that the patients are improving, but is that enough? Are we doing this only to comply with the regulatory agencies? While agencies are certainly a driving force, we have an opportunity to turn this activity into a process that can work for and with us. Since we know that it costs less to provide quality care right the first time, why not spend our time and energy determining the right way to do something and then do it right?

In addition, with the current environment of competition between home health providers, quality of care and the clear proof of that quality often becomes a significant determining factor in the selection of a home health provider. As our patients become more aware of their rights and responsibilities in relation to the selection of their health care providers, we can no longer rely upon linkages for established referral sources.

Home care organizations are having to "earn" the right to receive referrals. Managed care companies are expecting a high quality outcome at a minimum of cost. We need to consider the following components of quality:

> Quality is a long, ongoing process; to succeed, hospice and home care organizations can use information and learn from both quality assurance and quality improvement efforts. Quality is a challenge that takes time and must be done a step at a time throughout all levels of an organization within the confines of a restrictive legislative environment. A commitment to quality pays off, as many success stories in the health care field demonstrate—it is a process that benefits

the entire organization and the patients it serves. From a financial perspective, quality could 'save your hide.' From the regulatory perspective, quality isn't just a good idea any more—it's the law. (*Joint Commission on Accreditation of Healthcare Organizations*, 1990, p. 91)

The purpose of this chapter is to expose occupational therapy practitioners in home health to quality management concepts and terms, so they in turn may feel greater comfort in participating in quality management activities in their agencies. Through this participation, occupational therapists and occupational therapy assistants can assure, in a measurable and scientific manner, that their services are effective, while educating others on the perspective and value that occupational therapy has to offer. To be a part of the process of measuring quality is an important force in guaranteeing the profession's place in the health care community of providers.

The content of the chapter is presented in an order designed to address both the concepts of quality management and the application of these concepts in a practice setting. Specific examples of areas for monitoring are listed later in this chapter.

II. Organizations That Measure Quality in Home Health

Much of this chapter is focused on the Joint Commission on Accreditation of Healthcare Organizations (JCAHO), a national accreditation body whose standards and guidelines have been a significant force in the move toward measuring quality of care. However, it is also important to note the work of other organizations. The Health Care Financing Administration (HCFA) has provided guidance in the form of Generic Quality Screens to assess the quality of care provided in the home. These screens are related to such areas as adequacy and timeliness of intake, evaluation, and intervention; infections; documented follow-up planning; and any events or patterns of care resulting in adverse outcomes. All Medicare-certified home health agencies must meet or exceed the expectations of these quality screens to achieve or maintain their Medicare participation for reimbursement. In addition, many states have their own quality guidelines that home health agencies must meet in order to achieve or maintain state licensure.

An alternative to JCAHO accreditation that many home care organizations pursue is that of the Community Health Accreditation Program, Inc. (CHAP). CHAP is a subsidiary of the National

League for Nursing. CHAP's purpose is to elevate the quality of home care in this country and to counter public fears about a quality crisis in this increasingly crucial health care arena. The CHAP standards concerning quality require the organization to consistently provide high quality services and products through the following ways:

- An emphasis on quality emanating from philosophy and purpose statements including the strategic plan, staff orientation and development programs, and staff familiarity with the organizational commitment.
- Services and products that are accessible and available to clients.
- Effective intraorganizational coordination.
- Organizational policies and procedures developed for all programs.
- Service records maintained for each client, or client group, for coordination; legal documentation; and meeting reimbursement requirements.
- Adequacy, appropriateness, and effectiveness of services and products that is routinely assessed and measured to assure high quality. Findings are utilized to improve quality.

Within the specific CHAP standard regarding evaluation of quality (Standard CII.6.), the following are considered (Brown, 1993):

- The quality assurance plan identifies goals and purposes, standards and criteria, descriptions of processes including time frame and individual responsibilities, and mechanisms for a follow-up of findings.
- Quality assurance measures include these characteristics at minimum: client outcome data, client satisfaction evaluation, clinical record reviews, peer reviews, and program evaluations.
- Results of all the quality assessment activities are used as a basis for resolving identified problems, improving the quality of services and products, and making needed changes. All are used in the planning process.
- Quality of services is defined and measured in terms of client outcomes. Measurable client-outcome program objectives for each program identify recipients of service, expected behavior or result of service, time frame for expected results, and percentage of recipients realistically expected to demonstrate results within expected time frame.

- Client and caregiver satisfaction with services and products is routinely monitored, evaluated, and considered in assessing the quality of services and products; and developing strategies for improvement of services, program planning, and evaluation including satisfaction with services, staff, and with a client's own participation in care.
- Understanding of and agreement with cause and timeliness of cessation of care. This includes understanding the organization's Client Bill of Rights, and suggestions for improvement of specific complaints.
- Service records are systematically reviewed in order to determine the appropriateness and adequacy of service, as well as compliance with established policies regarding client care and professional practice.
- Representatives of each discipline are routinely involved in the evaluation of the quality of care delivered by that discipline and make recommendations based on their findings.

III. Background History of the Quest for Quality: The Joint Commission's Role

While most of us prefer to operate in the here and now, it is helpful to gain a perspective on the evolutionary process that has occurred as health care systems attempt to define and quantify quality. Since specific home care organizations may utilize a variety of quality management techniques, an overview of this process may be useful.

Historically, the quest for quality in health care in our country has been reflected in the evolution through various stages; most recently through JCAHO and other accrediting and regulatory bodies. At first, the emphasis was on implicit review (morbidity and mortality review). This then grew into time-limited studies (retrospective audits) and gradually into ongoing monitoring and evaluation (Quality Assurance or QA). It is notable, however, that as these expansions occurred, some elements of the previous criteria were retained as necessary and helpful. This trend continues as the best of each function is retained.

One of the most significant contributions JCAHO made to the clarification of quality assurance was the Ten-Step Process for Monitoring and Evaluation, as graphically outlined in Figure 1 on page 78.

As JCAHO's "Agenda for Change" (a term employed during the transition from Quality Assurance to Quality Improvement) progressed, the 1992 evolution from Quality Assurance to Continuous Quality Improvement shifted the focus to an increased awareness of the need to demonstrate the quality of care provided. As summarized by Higgins (AOTA, 1994), JCAHO modified the elements that distinguished the quality improvement concepts from the traditional quality assurance methods in the following ways:
- A focus on the process of creating a product or service; not the people providing the service.
- A definition of quality that meets the needs of the customer (e.g., patients, families, physicians, payers, suppliers, and health care providers).
- An improvement in quality that results in a reduction in costs.
- A strategy of building quality into the process, not by the use of end inspections alone.
- A scientific approach to problem solving (e.g., multidisciplinary teams and statistical methods).
- A view of quality as a management strategy that crosses traditional boundaries.

Changing this focus involved greater depth in assessing what the "customers" (as noted above) wanted to see in a quality organization. This required the addition of several significant components. In the Ten-Step Monitoring and Evaluation Process (see Figure 1) enhancements were made to Step 6 regarding the collection and organization of data. Currently, feedback is requested from all types of customers, not simply the patients. For instance, insurance companies and referral sources collect feedback data through surveys, comments, suggestions, and complaints. The emphasis is on organizations gaining input from a variety of sources.

This shift was demonstrated in the 1992 modifications to JCAHO's Ten-Step Process for Monitoring and Evaluation as evidenced in Figure 2 on page 79.

Although the focus in the evolution of quality management is moving toward improving organizational performance through consideration of key functions within the provision of services, there is still a need for quality evaluation through monitoring and evaluation techniques. One method for accomplishing this activity is through the JCAHO's Ten-Step Process noted in Figure 2. The following is an outline of the entire process:

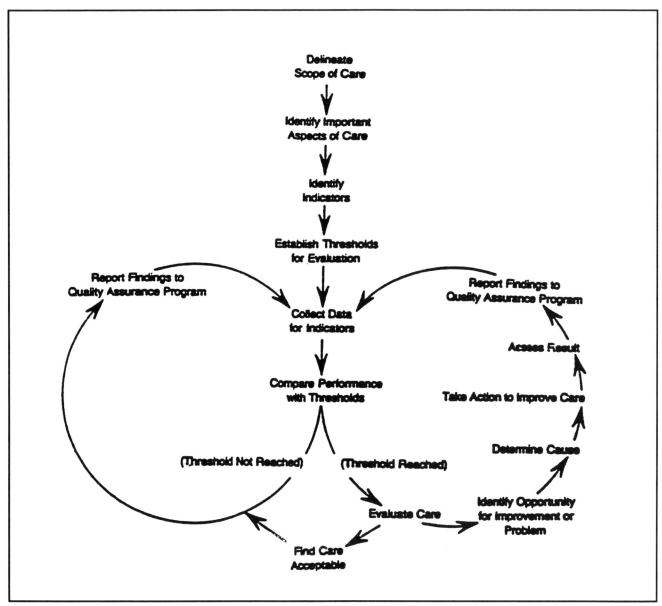

FIGURE 1: JCAHO'S TEN-STEP PROCESS FOR MONITORING AND EVALUATION)

Reprinted with permission from *Quality Assurance in Home Care and Hospice Organizations* (p. 43) by the Joint Commission on Accreditation of Healthcare Organizations, 1990, Oakbrook Terrace, IL: Author.

Step 1.

Assign Responsibility

a. Involve organization leaders.

b. Design and foster approach to continuous improvement of quality.

c. Set priorities for evaluation and improvement.

Step 2.

Delineate Scope of Care and Service

a. Identify key functions and/or identify the procedures, treatments, and other activities performed in the organization.

Step 3.

Identify Important Aspects of Care and Service

a. Determine the key functions, treatments, processes, and other aspects of care and service that warrant ongoing monitoring.

b. Establish priorities among the important aspects of care and service chosen.

Step 4.

Identify Indicators

a. Identify teams to develop indicators for the important aspects of care and service.

b. Select indicators.

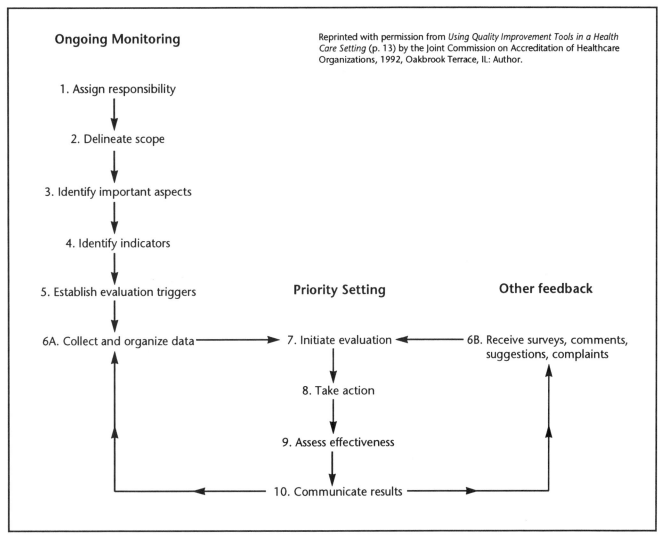

Ongoing Monitoring

Reprinted with permission from *Using Quality Improvement Tools in a Health Care Setting* (p. 13) by the Joint Commission on Accreditation of Healthcare Organizations, 1992, Oakbrook Terrace, IL: Author.

1. Assign responsibility

2. Delineate scope

3. Identify important aspects

4. Identify indicators

5. Establish evaluation triggers

Priority Setting

Other feedback

6A. Collect and organize data → 7. Initiate evaluation ← 6B. Receive surveys, comments, suggestions, complaints

8. Take action

9. Assess effectiveness

10. Communicate results

FIGURE 2: 1992 MODIFICATIONS TO JCAHO'S TEN-STEP PROCESS.

Step 5.

Establish a Means to Trigger Evaluation

a. For each indicator, the team identifies how evaluation may be triggered.

b. Select the means to trigger evaluation.

Step 6.

Collect and Organize Data

a. Each team identifies data sources and data-collection methods for the recommended indicators.

b. Design the final data-collection methodology, including those responsible for collecting, organizing, and determining whether evaluation is triggered.

c. Collect data.

d. Organize data to determine whether evaluation is required.

e. Collect data from other sources, including patient and staff surveys, comments, suggestions, and complaints.

Step 7.

Initiate Evaluation

a. Determine whether evaluation should be initiated.

b. Assess other feedback (for example, staff suggestions, patient-satisfaction survey results) that may contribute to priority setting for evaluation.

c. Set priorities for evaluation.

d. Teams undertake intensive evaluation.

Step 8.

Take Actions to Improve Care and Service

a. Teams recommend and/or take actions.

Step 9.

Assess the Effectiveness of Actions and Ensure that Improvement is Maintained

a. Assess to determine whether care and service have improved.

b. If not, determine further action.

c. Repeat (a) and (b) until improvement is obtained and maintained.

d. Maintain monitoring.

e. Periodically reassess priorities for monitoring.

Step 10.

Communicate Results to Relevant Individuals and Groups

a. Teams forward conclusions, actions, and results to leaders and to affected individuals, committees, departments, and services.

b. Disseminate information as necessary.

c. Leaders and others receive and disseminate comments, reactions, and information from involved individuals and groups. (Joint Commission on Accreditation of Healthcare Organizations, 1992, p. 14)

IV. Changes From Quality Assurance to Continuous Quality Improvement

Two components were added in the evolution of continuous quality improvement; the first being the use of a multidisciplinary team approach to problem evaluation and problem solving, and the second was expanded use of statistical methods for data collection and organization. Both of these components are familiar to occupational therapy practitioners, as our background and training facilitates their use. Perhaps our greatest asset is in the area of the multidisciplinary teams, often called "Quality Teams" or "Quality Indicator Teams." Our training and expertise in the group process and group dynamics provides real insight into participation in, and often leadership of, this team process. The goal of the quality team is to bring experts (not just the department managers) together to study an issue or process that relates to patient care, crossing the traditional departmental and organizational boundaries. These experts represent those individuals most involved in or aware of the process being considered.

The use of statistical methods enhances this team concept. These methods have the advantage of being "clean" in that they can pinpoint the root cause or situation from a range of variables. In addition, statistics can provide a clear and concise presentation of information through visual displays such as graphs and flow charts. These tools enable the team process to proceed rapidly and effectively. For example, the use of a flow chart can assist the occupational therapy practitioner in determining a trouble spot in the flow of referrals to the service, or in timely completion of evaluations. More information on the application of statistical tools is available from a variety of sources, particularly *The Memory Jogger* by Goal/QPC, listed in the suggested readings.

After JCAHO's initial "push" toward the move to continuous quality improvement as a means to move an organization toward the corporate culture of Total Quality Management (TQM), JCAHO backed off on mandating the use of any specific method. Instead the organization required that there must be evidence of a focus on continual improvement. This evidence should reflect that any organization is aware of the need for the following:

- Continually measuring the stability of systems and processes (e.g., statistical quality control, or any other method of analyzing data collected).
- Utilizing outcome measurements in determining priorities for improving systems and processes.
- Creating awareness of individual competence and performance.

As JCAHO's focus evolved into the 1994 hospital standards, the shift was toward improving organizational performance. The first evidence of this change was in the 1994 hospital manual that was reorganized into four major sections. These areas related to: Care of the Patient, Organizational Functions, Structures with Important Functions, and Other Department/Service Specific Requirements. This change reflected the focal shift from department-specific to overall organizational function and performance orientation. The intent was to cross traditional departmental lines and explore those key functions that involve interdisciplinary cooperation and coordination.

Many of the categories within these key functions relate directly to home health occupational therapy; particularly those relating to the evaluation of patients, treatment of patients, and patient/family education. While previous monitoring activities were concerned with three areas (structure, process, and outcome), the emphasis had now shifted to a primary focus on process and particularly outcome of patient care, with structure being looked at as "quality control." Quality control relates to those areas needing to be monitored in order to assure quality care was provided, but not relating to more than one specific discipline. Examples of this process might include the completeness of the occupational therapy evaluation, or monitoring the skin condition after an application of a hand splint. In this conceptual framework, the traditional Ten-Step Monitoring is no longer required but the standards do require that some sort of process is in place to systematically measure the quality of care provided.

In addition, a process from JCAHO, first presented in the 1994 hospital standards manual, provides guidance in terms of addressing key functional processes inclusive of the quality evaluation monitoring and evaluation. The flow chart in Figure 3 illustrates the process for improving performance and outcomes in a health care organization (see Figure 3). It is similar to the PDCA (Plan-Do-Check-Act) process familiar to many therapists. For further explanation of this type of process, see page 17 of the JCAHO book entitled *Using Quality Improvement Tools in a Health Care Setting* noted in the references and suggested readings.

Based on the 1994 JCAHO hospital standards and the Joint Commission's overall restructuring of its accreditation standards for all programs, it can be assumed that the quality management standards of the 1995 home care standards will include the following components:

- Structure that reflects a planned, systematic, organization-wide approach to the design, measurement, evaluation, and improvement of performance that is accomplished in a collaborative manner and includes all necessary services and disciplines.

- Processes that are well-designed and based on the organization's mission, vision, and plan so that the needs and expectations of patients, staff, and others are addressed in such a manner that utilizes current sources of information in the form of practice guidelines/parameters, and addresses performance compared to other organizations via reference databases.

- Measurement that is accomplished through a systematic process of data collection that includes the following: attention to both processes and outcomes; activities relating to both prioritized improvement issues and continuing measurement; addressing perfor-

FIGURE 3: FRAMEWORK FOR IMPROVEMENT.

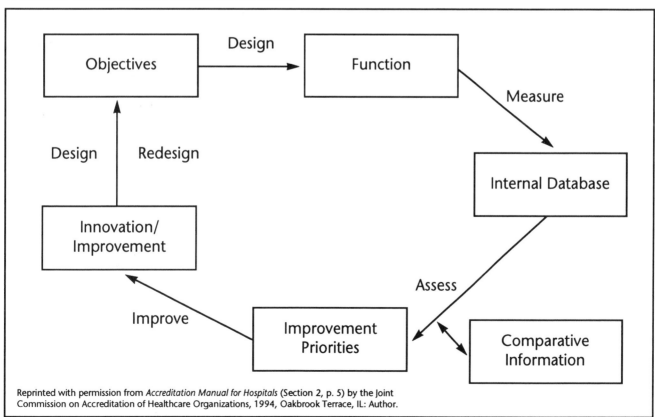

Reprinted with permission from *Accreditation Manual for Hospitals* (Section 2, p. 5) by the Joint Commission on Accreditation of Healthcare Organizations, 1994, Oakbrook Terrace, IL: Author.

mance that meets the needs and expectations of patients, staff and others; encompassing all key organizational functions, particularly those that represent a high volume of patients that place them at serious risk if not performed well, performed when not indicated, or are likely to be problem prone.

- Quality control activity data, if applicable, must be assessed in at least the areas of clinical laboratory services, equipment provided to patients, and equipment used in treating patients.
- Evaluation of the data collected must be done utilizing a systematic process including: statistical quality control techniques; comparison data that reflects processes and outcomes over time and comparisons to practice guidelines/parameters and other organizations through use of databases; evaluation of variation that focuses on performance when triggered by important single events, significant differences from other organizations, or accepted standards or opportunities to improve; and, if a need is demonstrated relative to individual competency issues, action is taken.
- Actions taken will be through a systematic process of identifying improvement priorities considering key functions, required resources, and the relationship to the organization's mission. Activity will consider the impact on performance including both expectations and measures of performance, and will involve appropriate individuals and departments/services. Action may be trial tested, with modifications as necessary, before overall implementation.

V. Definitions

The standards indicated above include many references to "dimensions of performance." It is expected that a focus on the performance of functions will be reflected in both the patient outcomes and the cost of the services provided.

JCAHO defines these dimensions in the following manner:

Doing the Right Thing:

- The *efficacy* of the procedure or treatment in relation to the patient's condition: The degree to which the care/intervention for the patient has been shown to accomplish the desired/projected outcome(s).

- The *appropriateness* of a specific test, procedure, or service to meet the patient's needs: The degree to which the care/intervention provided is relevant to the patient's clinical needs, given the current state of knowledge.

Doing the Right Thing Well:

- The *availability* of a needed test, procedure, treatment, or service to the patient who needs it: The degree to which appropriate care/intervention is available to meet the patient's needs.

- The *timeliness* with which a needed test, procedure, treatment, or service is provided to the patient: The degree to which the care/intervention is provided to the patient at the most beneficial or necessary time.

- The *effectiveness* with which tests, procedures, treatments, and services are provided: The degree to which the care/intervention is provided in the correct manner, given the current state of knowledge, in order to achieve the desired/projected outcome for the patient.

- The *continuity* of the services provided to the patient with respect to other services, practitioners, and providers and over time: The degree to which the care/intervention for the patient is coordinated among practitioners, among organizations, and over time.

- The *safety* of the patient (and others) to whom the services are provided: the degree to which the risk of an intervention and the risk in the care environment are reduced for the patient and others, including the health care provider.

- The *efficiency* with which services are provided: The relationship between the outcomes (results of care) and the resources used to deliver patient care.

- The *respect and caring* with which services are provided: The degree to which the patient or a designated individual is involved in his/her own care decisions and to which those providing services do so with sensitivity and respect for the patient's needs, expectations, and individual differences. (Joint Commission on Accreditation of Healthcare Organizations, 1994, Section 2, p. 2)

These definitions reach to the heart of the performance of occupational therapy in any setting, but particularly in the home health setting. This terminology is useful in focusing our documentation of need for services and value of those services provided. The use of these specific terms can assist both the new and experienced practitioners in verbalizing the quality of care provided. This reference range also provides the possible base for incorporating quality management information into competency ratings, performance evaluations, and the evaluation of continuing education needs, as this requirement is clear in the standard for action taken relative to specific practitioners. These performance dimensions can even be used in development of parameters for outcomes research.

In addition, the following definitions of specific quality management terms from the Joint Commission's *Accreditation Manual for Hospitals* (1994) will help therapists to be aware of the current use of these terms as they relate to descriptions of quality:

assess: To transform data into information by analyzing the data.

criteria: Expected level(s) of achievement, or specifications against which performance can be assessed.

improve: To take actions that result in the desired measurable change in the identified performance dimension.

indicator: A tool used to measure, over time, the performance of functions, processes, and outcomes of an organization.

measure: To collect quantified data about a dimension of performance of a function or process.

measurement: The systematic process of data collection, repeated over time or at a single point in time.

organization-wide: Throughout the organization and across multiple structural and staffing components, as appropriate.

outcome: The result of the performance (or nonperformance) of a function or process(es).

performance measure: A measure, such as a standard or indicator, used to assess the performance of a function or process of any organization.

plan: To formulate/describe the approach to achieving the goals related to improving the performance of the organization.

process: A goal-directed, interrelated series of actions, events, mechanisms, or steps.

reference database: An organized collection of similar data from many organizations that can be used to compare an organization's performance to that of others.

relevant: Having a clearly decisive bearing on an issue.

sentinel event: An occurrence that, when noted, requires intensive evaluation.

systematic: Pursuing a defined objective(s) in a planned, step-by-step manner.

variance: A measure of the differences in a set of observations.

variation: The differences in results obtained in measuring the same phenomenon more than once. The sources of variation in a process over time can be grouped into two major classes—common causes and special causes. (Joint Commission on Accreditation of Healthcare Organizations, 1994, Section 2, p. 4–5)

In an attempt to summarize the evolution of quality management over the past several decades, Higgins (AOTA, 1994) has provided the following overview. Each addition or improvement is built upon the strengths of the previous activity, therefore the overview is modeled from the bottom up, and should be read in that manner (see Figure 4).

FIGURE 4: EVOLUTION OF QUALITY MANAGEMENT.

Improving Organizational Performance (IOP):
Focus shifts to organization-wide performance of key functional areas
Addressing the dimensions of performance
Quality assurance changes to quality assessment
Focus shifts to outcomes
Emphasis on outcomes research
Benchmarking for comparisons regarding performance
Multidisciplinary shifts to interdisciplinary

Continuous Quality Improvement (CQI):
Quality assurance monitoring and evaluation enhanced (including opportunities for improvement)
Other forms of input added to traditional monitoring and evaluation
Customer satisfaction (internal and external) driven
Quality teams-oriented toward processes
Utilization of statistical tools
Shift away from individual performance to groups performing well
Desire for multidisciplinary monitoring activities

Quality Assurance (QA):
Monitoring and evaluation including concurrent reviews
Attempts to create change while the patient is in the system
Equal balance of orientation toward structure, process, and outcome
Focus on identifying individual outliers

Chart Audits:
Retrospective reviews addressing correct usage of resources
oriented toward structure over process and outcome

Adapted from *AOTA QI Resource Guide* (p. 131) by the American Occupational Therapy Association, 1994, Rockville, MD: Author.

VI. Methodology

To this point, an overview of the history of and rationale for quality management in home health occupational therapy have been presented. Many therapists may respond by asking "So, how do I do it?" While there are no "cookbook" answers or outlines that will work for all organizations, there are some common themes and components to consider. Keeping in mind the dimensions of performance previously indicated, focus on those key functions that involve the provision of occupational therapy services within your organizational framework.

Practitioners new to these concepts may be able to add their monitoring needs to an existing activity within the agency through such areas as patient satisfaction surveys or interdisciplinary tracking of the timeliness and completeness of documentation. The easiest monitoring can be done on functional outcomes. For example, functional outcome studies can focus on selected patients increasing their independence in dressing skills, mobility, and meal preparation. Monitoring activities can be accomplished as simply as developing a checklist or graph that plots progress over time.

The following is a list, by no means inclusive of all possibilities, that highlights some areas to consider. When addressing these areas, therapists should work toward interdisciplinary monitoring activities that cross traditional departmental boundaries. Some of them can be addressed as "quality control" monitoring activities specifically within the occupational therapy service or department. Others will be "quality indicators" (those issues relating to several departments) generating a "quality team" or opportunity to improve organizational performance, as well as departmental performance.

- Treatment plan is appropriate, and goals and objectives are coordinated.

- Interdisciplinary team members are involved in rehabilitation care planning.

- Home health professional personnel comply with policies and procedures.

- Referrals are timely and appropriate.

- Patient/client is satisfied with the therapist.

- Scheduled treatments are carried out.

- Patient's/client's functional status is maintained or improved (i.e., mobility, independence, and alertness).

- Infection control policies and procedures are followed.

- Home health professional services personnel ensure the safety of patients/ clients while performing their duties (i.e., evaluation of patient/client incidents).

- Patient/client understands and complies with treatment plan. (Joint Commission on Accreditation of Healthcare Organizations, 1990, p. 131)

The above listings would be considered quality indicators since they are related to the activities of more than one discipline; not exclusively the occupational therapy service. If the home health agency is not addressing these in a comprehensive manner, they could be monitored within the occupational therapy department as a quality control monitor specific to that service.

In many smaller home health agencies, rehabilitation services may be staffed through a separate contracting organization. Quality management activities are still required to be conducted. The responsibility for this activity should be delineated in the contract between the agency and the staffing entity.

In addition to the preceeding list, practitioners should consider some of the following specific areas:

- Efficacy of adaptive or corrective equipment, and its safe application, cleaning, maintenance, and storage.
- Supervision of home health aides, both in terms of content of services and timeliness of interventions.
- Appropriateness of level of care or service.
- Family participation in discharge planning process.
- All aspects of communication within the treatment team.
- Documentation standards of the organization and local regulatory agencies.

The methodology of the monitoring of these processes and patient care outcomes becomes another unique factor in the home care setting. The obvious method is abstraction from the chart as the record of care, and this can prove very useful for a variety of retrospective monitoring activities. Information regarding overall trends will also be available in this manner. It is important, however, to also assess the performance of provision of care on an ongoing concurrent basis, so that immediate action can be taken to change the provision of care to specific patients if appropriate.

The home care setting presents challenges in this evaluation. In a 1994 article by Deborah Williams, OTR/L (Williams, 1994), she references the uniqueness in supervision of home care occupational therapy practitioners and the monitoring of their performance. Some of the considerations apply to other quality monitoring as well. Williams references both direct and indirect methods, including on-site visits and the peer review process. During on-site visits, key areas include: patient dynamics (active listening, focus on patient priorities); evaluation skills (initial evaluation, clear documentation of findings); patient/caretaker education (including comprehension); documentation (timeliness and treatment); time management (schedule coordinated with other services); and appropriateness of treatment (relationship to the plan and diagnosis). Peer review relates to a therapist's performance compared to agency and department-wide standards.

Last, but by no means least, is the consideration of other forms of input, most notably through patient and family satisfaction surveys, evaluation of patient complaints, and feedback from referring physicians.

VII. Components of a Complete Quality Management Program

In a broad context, a complete quality management program requires a blend of quality evaluation (formerly called *quality assurance*, with its familiar monitoring and evaluation process) and aspects of both risk management and utilization review. Just as occupational therapists cannot function in a vacuum without the rest of the home health team, quality management interrelates with these other essential functions.

As patients are discharged from an inpatient setting much earlier in their care process with the need for increasingly complex procedures, the potential risk factors facing the therapist in a home health setting increases significantly. While traditionally our risk areas have related to improving staff skills, preventing patient injuries, and dealing with incidents, now the therapist is faced with many of the complex risk situations before associated with inpatient therapy. Areas of risk that an occupational therapist should consider include:

- Occurrences/incidents that should be reported.
- Participation in an effective reporting system.
- Inclusion of occupational therapy components in a clear database of patient incidents, adverse outcomes of care, and patient injuries for the agency.
- Evaluation of the elements of risk within the occupational therapy activities.
- Development and provision of training and education of staff to reduce hazards.
- Training patients and families in their responsibilities.
- Development of security precautions as needed.
- Evaluation of equipment taken into the home by the therapist for both its safety and efficiency.

Awareness of risk factors is particularly difficult in the home setting, as the time spent by the therapist in the home is such a small percentage of the patient's total time, making supervision of equipment use difficult. This makes the education of the patient and family members essential in providing for safety. Some specific risk areas to consider include, but should not be limited to:

- Unclear referral orders.
- Improper use of equipment by patients.
- Incorrect application of equipment by family members.
- Skin breakdown with splints.
- Inadequate services provided by a contracted service.
- Lack of coordination/communication with the treatment team regarding increased risk factors either relating to the patient or the home environment.

Situations occurring which pose either a direct or an indirect risk should be communicated immediately through the organization's reporting mechanism, to other team members, and tracked for trend areas within the occupational therapy section. Clear and complete reporting of risk situations and incidents should feed directly into the quality management program as potential safety monitoring activities or the need for an interdisciplinary team to assess a process that may be adversely impacting patient outcomes.

Another function contributing to the quality management program is that of utilization review. JCAHO defines this type of review as one that "...functions to evaluate, against objective criteria, how well professional care, services, procedures, equipment and interventions are being employed in the proper setting to provide high-quality and cost-effective patient care" (Joint Commission on Accreditation of Healthcare Organizations, 1990, p. 21). When related to occupational therapy, emphasis is placed on the use of both occupational therapists and occupational therapy assistants within the organization, as well as supervision of home health aides. Specific guidelines regarding the level of care required for professional intervention and the supervision of support services staff (e.g., homemakers and companions), must be in place within the organization.

Clear and objective documentation by the practitioner is an essential part of enabling utilization review to take place. A complete and comprehensive evaluation of the patient by an occupational therapist may be the determining factor in approval of services, both by the referring physician and the funding source. Decisions for continued provision of services frequently hinges on the documentation by practitioners. The occupational therapy practitioner's involvement in the overall plan of comprehensive services for the patient is essential in determining the appropriate level of care that can be provided in the least restrictive setting. Therefore, the therapist must be aware of and planning toward discharge of the patient to follow-thorough by other services or resources (i.e., volunteers or family members).

VIII. Conclusion

While quality management is not the primary responsibility of the occupational therapy practitioner in the home health setting, it is an important consideration. Awareness of the current standards under which an organization functions, and the relationship of the occupational therapy section or department to which those standards are essential. Understanding of the basics and cooperation with the quality management staff can facilitate the influx of vital and useful information regarding the quality of care provided by the practitioner. In this era of rapidly changing standards and expectations, keeping our basics of quality care in mind can help to focus and clarify our role within the health care system.

In addition to the quality management activities described in this chapter, it must be noted that many home health occupational therapy practitioners may also be involved with other related aspects of measuring quality. For instance, an agency affiliated with an inpatient setting may include home health components of a clinical (or critical) pathway or practice parameters guiding the specifics of care provided in each phase of patient care. In this setting, the practitioner may need to address the transition of care from the acute phase to the home health setting to participate in the pathway. Today, some home health agencies are developing their own clinical/critical pathways that track a patient within their own system based on diagnoses.

In other situations, practitioners may be asked to participate in outcomes research or studies relative to the overall continuum of care of the patient. These present exciting and positive opportunities for growth and progress within the professional role of the practitioner, but they also require further study and enhancement of skills.

References

American Occupational Therapy Association. (1994). *AOTA QI Resource Guide*. Rockville, MD: Author.

Brown, J.A. (1993). *The Quality Management Professional's Study Guide*. Pasadena, CA: Managed Care Consultants.

Joint Commission Accreditation of Healthcare Organizations. (1994). *Accreditation Manual for Hospitals*. Oakbrook Terrace, IL: Author.

Joint Commission on Accreditation of Healthcare Organizations. (1992). *Using Quality Improvement Tools In A Health Care Setting*. Oakbrook Terrace, IL: Author.

Joint Commission on Accreditation of Healthcare Organizations. (1990). *Quality Assurance in Home Care and Hospice Organizations*. Oakbrook Terrace, IL: Author.

Williams, D. (1994). Supervision: Keeping track of treatment performed off site. *OT Week, 8*(3),17–18.

Suggested Readings

American Occupational Therapy Association. (1994). *AOTA QI Resource Guide*. Rockville, MD: Author.

Bassard, M. (1989). *The memory jogger plus*. Methuen, MA: Goal/QPC.

Berwick, D., Godfrey, A., & Roessner, J. (1990). *Curing health care*. San Francisco: Jossey-Bass.

Ciccone, K., & Lord, J. (1992). *Continuous performance improvement through integrated quality assessment*. Chicago: American Hospital.

Goal/QPC. (1988). *The memory jogger: A pocket guide of tools for continuous improvement*. Methuen, MA: Author.

JCAHO Publications—Available from JCAHO, One Renaissance Blvd., Oakbrook Terrace, IL 60181. Phone: (708) 916-5800.

- *A compendium of forms, tables, and charts for use in monitoring and evaluation*. (1991).
- *An introduction to quality improvement in health care*. (1991).
- *Exploring quality improvement principles: A hospital leader's guide*. (1992).
- *How to prepare for a survey: Physical rehabilitation services*. (1992).
- *Implementing quality improvement: A hospital leader's guide*. (1993).
- *Primer on indicator development and application measuring quality in health care*. (1990).
- *Quality assurance in home care and hospice organizations*. (1990).

- *The transition from QA to QI: Performance-based evaluation of mental health organizations.* (1992).
- *Using quality improvement tools in a health care setting.* (1992).

Joe, B. (Ed.), Lawlor, M., Scott, T., & Thien, M. (1991). *Quality assurance in occupational therapy: A practitioner's guide to setting up a QA system using three models.* Rockville, MD: American Occupational Therapy Association.

Juran, J. (1988). *Juran on planning for quality.* New York: Free Press.

Leebov, W., & Ersoz, C. (1991). *The health care manager's guide to continuous quality improvement.* Chicago. American Hospital.

Meisenheimer, C. (1989). *Quality assurance for home health care.* Gaithersburg, MD: Aspen Publishers.

Scholtes, P. (1988). *The team handbook.* Madison, WI: Joiner Associates.

Walton, M. (1988). *The Deming management method.* New York: Perigee.

Chapter 10
Discontinuation of Services

by Jennifer A. Young, COTA/L

I. Introduction

The discharge process of occupational therapy services in the home differs greatly from that of the hospital-based setting. In an acute care or rehab setting, the patient is automatically discharged because of diagnosis-related group (DRG) time lines. In the home, the practitioner has an active role in determining when the discharge is appropriate.

The discharge plan should begin at the initial visit and should include the family as well as the patient. The patient and the family should be made aware that discharge will occur when therapeutic goals are met or the patient is no longer homebound. Discharge might also occur because the insurance company has limited the number of visits. It is important that the patient is aware of these factors. With patients being discharged from the hospital sooner and with increased functional limitations ("GAO Study," 1985), it is important that the patient does not expect home health therapy to be a magical cure. Goals need to be realistic, measurable, and specific, with ongoing input from the patient and family.

II. Monitoring/Evaluation Under Medicare Part A Before Discharge

Medicare now allows reimbursement for monitoring and evaluation of the effectiveness of the maintenance program's activities. The nurse or the practitioner must document that the patient needs maintenance services to maintain the current level of functional ability. Services and their frequency must be justified for monitoring and evaluation. The practitioner might need to educate the fiscal intermediary to obtain reimbursement for these procedures.

III. Reasons for Discharge

As stated previously, discharge usually occurs when the patient has reached maximum potential within terms of functional performance. It can also occur if the patient is no longer homebound. The need for outpatient therapy may then be justified. Discharge may also occur when the fiscal intermediary or the private insurance company will no longer reimburse for services. Therefore, some agencies may discharge a patient from their services because of a visit reimbursement denial. (See Chapter 12 for more information on denials.)

IV. Standards of Practice for Occupational Therapy

Standard VIII of the American Occupational Therapy Association's (AOTA) *Standards of Practice for Occupational Therapy* (AOTA, 1994), refers to discharge of service in occupational therapy practice. These same guidelines can be followed in the home health setting. The following is the information that is included in Standard VIII:

Standard VIII: Discontinuation

1. A registered occupational therapist shall discontinue service when the individual has achieved predetermined goals or has achieved maximum benefit from occupational therapy services.

2. A registered occupational therapist, with input from a certified occupational therapy assistant where applicable, shall prepare and implement a discharge plan that is consistent with occupational therapy goals, individual goals, interdisciplinary team goals, family goals, and expected outcomes. The discharge plan shall address appropriate community resources for referral for psychosocial, cultural, and socioeconomic barriers and limitations that may need modification.

3. A registered occupational therapist shall document the changes between the initial and current states of functional ability and deficit in performance areas, performance components, and performance contexts. A certified occupational therapy assistant may contribute to the process under the supervision of a registered occupational therapist.

4. An occupational therapy practitioner shall allow sufficient time for the coordination and effective implementation of the discharge plan.

5. A registered occupational therapist shall document recommendations for follow-up or reevaluation when applicable. (AOTA, 1994, pp. 1039–1043)

V. The Discharge Process

The discharge process should be ongoing, beginning with the initial visit. When appropriate, the occupational therapist and the occupational therapy assistant should collaborate on the discharge plan. It is necessary to inform the referring physician of plans to discontinue direct treatment. At this time, the occupational therapist can state the outcomes of the intervention and describe the current functional and physical status of the

patient. Because the physician must be informed of all changes in the patient's treatment plan, written approval is necessary to discharge the patient from occupational therapy. If the patient is going to be discharged before the end of the recertification period, verbal approval must be followed by written approval from the physician and must be written on the patient's chart. Sometimes the written approval might be done after the patient has already been discharged but this is not encouraged. Policies may vary according to the interpretations and the procedure of the fiscal intermediaries and the home health agencies, and should be clarified by the practitioner's employing or contracting agency.

Discharge planning should include the patient, other members of the treatment team, the family, and any appropriate community resources such as day care, senior, or community care centers. It is sometimes possible to begin to access community resources from the patient's home during the visit. The practitioner then has access to firsthand information from the family on the availability of services for the patient.

At the time of discharge, the occupational therapist should review with the patient, his or her home functional activity exercise program and update it as needed; reinforce home safety procedures; and observe and document the patient's ability to use adaptive equipment. A copy of the written home program should be placed in the patient's chart to satisfy Medicare. The occupational therapist will also need to complete a discharge evaluation. Check with your agency regarding particular policies.

VI. Readmission

A patient may be readmitted to occupational therapy if a new problem develops. Under Medicare guidelines, the therapist or nurse must contact the physician for new orders. The occupational therapist will then complete a new evaluation. Consider the following example:

A patient was discharged from occupational therapy secondary to reaching maximum potential, but was unable to complete tub transfers because of decreased mobility. Patient's functional mobility improved with the continuation of physical therapy and patient is now safe to begin tub transfers.

Under Medicare, a primary service such as nursing, physical therapy, or speech therapy needs to be in on the case for occupational therapy to reassess. With private insurance, the requirements vary with individual plans and should be clarified before occupational therapy services are initiated.

Patients can also be readmitted to the agency. After a recent hospitalization and a new diagnosis, the patient can be readmitted to the agency and can qualify for further therapeutic intervention.

VII. Conclusion

The discharge process may differ for home health care from that of hospital-based occupational therapy, allowing increased input from the patient, the family, or the caregiver. It is important that the practitioner have a thorough knowledge of community resources, Medicare, and other payor guidelines and agency policies to assist with the discharge process. The practitioner needs to prepare the patient for discharge and have realistic goals. The home health setting allows for the practitioner to see the patient excel in functional performance in their own environment. A successful discharge plan is one that the patient and the practitioner have reviewed together, and the goals of treatment have successfully offset the patient's deficits.

References

American Occupational Therapy Association. (1994). Standards of practice for occupational therapy. *American Journal of Occupational Therapy, 48* (11), 1039–1043.

GAO study of Medicare's prospective payment system flags potential hazards for older Americans. (1985, Spring). *Aging Reports,* p.1.

Suggested Reading

American Occupational Therapy Association. (1992). *Effective documentation for occupational therapy.* Rockville, MD: Author.

Chapter 11

Reimbursement for Home Health Services

by Mary Jane Youngstrom, MS, OTR,

with contributions by
Michael J. Steinhauer,
OTR, MPH, FAOTA

I. Introduction

A clear understanding of the guidelines for reimbursement of occupational therapy provided in the home will assist occupational therapy practitioners in their effort to provide quality care to individuals in this particular environment. Reimbursement guidelines may influence treatment by setting parameters for the length and/or type of service that will be covered. When the practitioner is aware of these parameters, decisions about treatment goals and services can be selected to best serve the patient within the limits allowed. Also, an awareness of reimbursement guidelines can assist practitioners in maintaining a positive relationship with third-party payers and fiscal intermediaries. Given the profession's continuing efforts to improve patient's and administrative personnel's awareness of occupational therapy, practitioners can more adequately discuss changes in reimbursement patterns as they affect the profession and the home health benefit as a whole. Occupational therapists and occupational therapy assistants are encouraged to have a broad-based knowledge of reimbursement principles, regardless of the specific payer, as well as specific information about individual payer's parameters for reimbursement. With such a background, practitioners can adjust to changes in coverage requirements with relative ease and minimize disruption of their practice and the services they provide to patients.

The information presented in this chapter is meant to provide a broad overview of reimbursement issues and practices in the home health arena and is aimed at assisting the practitioner in understanding the differences among the various kinds of coverage plans. It is not intended to reflect any of the most recent changes or regulatory differences among different states, intermediaries, or insurance companies. Occupational therapy practitioners are advised to directly confirm with their home health agency, intermediary, or third-party payer, the precise provisions for reimbursement for any particular plan or individual. The criteria for coverage and the limitations on services vary depending on the type of insurance plan and/or the individual policy. For example, private payers may limit the number of visits allowed within a specified time frame, whereas Medicare bases need for continuation of service on continuing functional change.

II. Medicare

Although home health services are a benefit provided in a variety of insurance plans, Medicare—the federal government's health insurance plan for the Social Security recipient over the age of 65 and the disabled—is by far the primary reimbursement source of home health benefits in the United States today. Familiarity with the Medicare rules and regulations is helpful because many other plans are patterned after them and often follow their lead.

Currently, Medicare insurance consists of two plans comprising Part A and Part B. Medicare Part A coverage is automatically provided for persons entitled to Medicare according to federal law. Part B is optional and must be paid for by the individual through monthly premium payments. Coverage under each part is summarized in Table 1. Note that Medicare Part A is designed to provide coverage for inpatient hospital services and services provided by other institutional providers such as nursing homes and home health agencies. Part B is aimed at providing coverage for services that an individual can access on an "outpatient" basis. Services are defined in terms of the specifics involved and may be furnished by individuals such as physicians, medical supply providers, and therapists.

Medicare Part A and B also differ in the way that they are billed and reimbursed. Institutional or individual providers must use different procedures and forms in billing for Medicare Part A and B. Reimbursement differs in that under Part A, Medicare will reimburse the provider 100% of the allowable charge but only 80% of the allowable charge under Part B. The remaining 20% must be billed to the individual patient or to the patient's supplementary insurance plan.

Although home health is a reimbursable service under both Medicare Part A and Part B, due to the differences in billing procedures and reimbursement formulas, most home health agencies do not choose to bill under both plans. The majority of agencies bill primarily under Part A. Individual occupational therapists working in their own private practice and who are certified as Medicare Part B providers, may bill under Part B but must follow all required billing and reimbursement procedures and will need to bill both Medicare and the patient.

To receive home health benefits under either Part A or Part B, prior hospitalization is not required. The number of home health visits are not limited arbitrarily but are dependent upon the

Part A Institutional Health Care Providers	Part B Specific Medical Services
Hospital inpatient (includes all therapies)	Physician's services
Skilled nursing facility—inpatient	Ambulance
Home health care	Durable medical equipment
Hospice	Facility-based outpatient services
	Individual certified providers of physical therapy, occupational therapy, and speech-language pathology provided in a variety of settings
	Home health care
	Many other health services and supplies (may be provided as an outpatient or while a resident is in a skilled nursing facility)

TABLE 1. GENERAL MEDICARE COVERAGE.

beneficiary's progress. Intermediaries do issue guidelines about visit frequencies, however, the guidelines are not meant to be restrictive.

The Health Care Financing Administration (HCFA) has established federal regulations for the Medicare system. The actual administration of the program and interpretation of the regulations are carried out by a designated fiscal intermediary (e.g., an insurance company chosen to represent Medicare). All home health agencies are assigned to one of ten regional intermediaries who have contracted with the government to carry out Medicare's business in a designated region. Significantly, intermediaries may differ in their interpretations and enforcement of federal/HCFA guidelines. For instance, what is accepted intermediary practice in California may not always be accepted intermediary practice in Texas. Consequently, familiarity with your own intermediary's guidelines and their interpretations is very important.

A. Eligibility Criteria

To be eligible for Part A home health benefits under Medicare, the following conditions must be met:

- Homebound—The patient does not have to be bedridden and, may even on infrequent occasions, leave the home such as for a physician's appointment. In general, homebound means that to leave the home requires considerable and taxing effort on the patient's part and the requires assistance of another person or device. (Also refer to Chapter 1, section on "Specifying the Term 'Homebound,'" p. 3.)
- Physician referral—The patient must be under the care of a physician who certifies that home health services are indicated.
- Requires skilled services—The patient is initially in need of physical therapy, speech-language pathology, or skilled nursing services on an intermittent basis.

Patients are eligible to receive home health benefits as long as the above criteria are met.

B. Criteria for Occupational Therapy Coverage

The need for occupational therapy alone does not initially qualify a patient for Part A home health services. Occupational therapy can, however, be introduced along with any one of the three initially qualifying services (nursing, physical therapy, speech-language pathology) and may continue once the other services have stopped. This does not mean that only one visit from a nurse, physical therapist, or speech-language pathologist is required to initiate occupational therapy. Cases in which an agency tries to make one visit meet the requirement tend to be more closely scrutinized by the intermediary because the need for intermittent treatment may not have been demonstrated. After the initial qualifying services have discontinued, the continuation of occupational therapy services is determined by the patient's individual need and progress.

Other criteria that must be met for occupational therapy to be covered includes the following elements:
- Treatment requires a specific physician's order for occupational therapy.
- Treatment must be performed by a qualified occupational therapist, or by a qualified occupational therapy assistant under the supervision of a qualified occupational therapist.
- Treatment must be reasonable and necessary for the patient's illness or injury.

The term "reasonable and necessary" is open to interpretation. Understanding how Medicare defines these terms can be helpful to the therapist because decisions about claim payment may be based on this interpretation. Some specific considerations that may be helpful in determining whether treatment is reasonable and necessary include the following:
- Treatment must result in significant practical improvement in functioning in a reasonably predictable amount of time based on diagnosis, severity, and prognosis.
- A valid expectation of improvement must exist at the time of evaluation although the expectation may not be realized.
- Necessity of treatment is based on demonstrating that the patient has a decrease in function. Any diagnosis could warrant occupational therapy intervention as long as a functional problem is demonstrated.
- There must be some demonstration of measurable and continuous improvement. Once a patient recovers or plateaus, treatment programs implemented to maintain function are not reimbursed. The skills of an occupational therapy practitioner will be reimbursed for the following: designing a maintenance program (1 to 2 visits generally will be covered); periodically reevaluating the maintenance program's effectiveness and changing or updating the program as necessary; and carrying out a maintenance program while training or retraining caregivers if there has been a change in the situation.

Refer to Chapter 8 on documentation for discussion and examples of how to document these criteria.

C. Covered Occupational Therapy Services

The Medicare benefit for occupational therapy includes coverage for the evaluation of referred patients as well as the planning, implementation, and supervision of therapeutic programs. Under the home health regulations, Medicare generally requires that evaluation and treatment occur within the same session. A session that included only evaluation services would be covered if its purpose was to determine the patient's need for skilled home health services and the need was substantiated. However, if the evaluation revealed that the need for skilled services was not supported, then the evaluation visit would not be reimbursed. Intermediary interpretation may vary on this issue. To ensure reimbursement, evaluation sessions should also document treatment services. In addition, Medicare will reimburse the patient for occupational therapist or occupational therapy assistant services, as appropriate, for the following:

- The design, fabrication, and fitting of orthotic and self-help devices.
- The provision of treatment oriented toward vocational and prevocational evaluation and training.

Patients with specifically diagnosed psychiatric illnesses may be reimbursed for occupational therapy treatment under home health (HCFA, 1989). However, Medicare differentiates between therapy for these diagnoses and therapy in the home solely to meet "motivational needs." Reimbursement is considered unlikely when the individual's therapeutic program is not directly and specifically related to a clearly identified, defined, and documented psychiatric illness and coexisting functional problems.

Medicare does, however, recognize the role of occupational therapy in treating the cognitive deficits associated with psychiatric and physical disabilities. The regulations issued by HCFA in 1990 clearly define the levels of assistance that can be used by practitioners to describe the patient's current functional status (see Chapter 8 on documentation for a thorough discussion). Each level defined (total, maximum, moderate, minimum, stand-by, and independent) includes a description of the individual's physical needs for assistance as well as the degree of cognitive assistance required (e.g., one-to-one demonstration, intermittent verbal cuing, or help in correcting mistakes) (HCFA, 1990). The inclusion of these cognitive parameters in Medicare's understanding of function more clearly defines occupational therapy's role in the treatment of individuals with psychiatric problems and those individuals with physical diagnoses complicated by cognitive deficits. Table 2 outlines the types and levels of physical and cognitive assistance that can be used to document change. Practitioner use of these descriptions can enhance reimbursement and more clearly articulate patient progress.

TABLE 2. LEVELS OF ASSISTANCE.

Assistance Level	Physical Assistance	Cognitive Assistance
Total	100% assistance by one or more persons to perform all physical activities.	External stimuli are required to elicit automatic actions such as swallowing.
Maximum	75% assistance by one person to physically perform any part of a functional activity.	Cognitive assistance such as 1:1 demonstration or sensory input is needed to perform gross motor actions in response to direction.
Moderate	50% assistance by one person to perform physical activities.	Constant cognitive assistance such as intermittent 1:1 demonstrations or physical or verbal cuing are needed to sustain and complete simple, repetitive tasks safely.
Minimum	25% assistance by one person for physical activities. Set up or help needed to initiate or sustain performance.	Periodic cognitive assistance is needed to correct repeated mistakes, check for safety compliance, or solve problems presented by unexpected hazards.
Stand-by	Supervision by one person to perform new procedure adapted by practitioner for safe and effective performance. Patient does not use safety precautions and demonstrates errors in performance.	
Independent	No physical assistance.	No cognitive assistance.

Table adapted from *Medicare Intermediary Manual, Part 3, Claims Process* (DHHS Transmittal No. 1487, Section 3906.4) by the Health Care Financing Administration, 1990, Washington, DC: U.S. Government Printing Office.

D. Supplies and Equipment

The costs of various supplies and equipment used in treatment to improve functioning (e.g., splinting materials, theraputty, or adaptive equipment used in demonstrations only) may be included in the occupational therapy cost center and are subject to reimbursement by Medicare only under the "General and Administrative Expenses" category. As an employee of a home health agency you would have access to these supplies and equipment. However, inventories are generally limited. As an independent contractor you probably would be responsible for providing your own.

Equipment that may be needed by the patient is considered in a separate category. Medicare will reimburse for durable medical equipment (DME) if:

- It meets the definition of DME; and if
- it is necessary and reasonable for the treatment of an illness or injury, or to improve functions of a malformed body member.

Medicare defines DME as equipment that: (bullet list)

- Can withstand repeated use;
- is primarily and customarily used to serve a medical purpose;
- generally is not useful to a person in the absence of illness or injury; and
- is appropriate for use in the home.

"Medical necessity" is a key term in Medicare's understanding of DME. Items that may be necessary for the patient's improved functioning, but are not medically necessary for the treatment of the patient's medical condition, are not reimbursable. Examples of covered and noncovered DME are outlined in Table 3. Items such are grab bars, raised toilet seats, and bath benches are considered convenience items, and are not directly related to treatment of the medical condition. They are therefore not considered to be medically necessary. Adaptive self-help equipment that occupational therapy practitioners often recommend are also not covered because they are not considered to be primarily medical in nature.

All claims for DME, prosthetics, orthotics, and supplies (DMEPOS) are submitted to Medicare through one of four regional carriers referred to at Durable Medical Equipment Regional Carriers (DMERCs). The DMERC processes the claim and payment. In the case of items that are not specifically included or excluded, the DMERC will review and rule on the medical necessity of DMEPOS. All suppliers of DMEPOS (i.e., medical equipment dealers, physicians, therapists in their own private practice) who provide DME, must have a supplier

Covered	Noncovered
Hospital bed	Grab bars
Wheelchairs	Toilet seats—raised
Trapeze bar—if confined to bed	Over-bed table
	Reachers
Commode—if confined to bed or room	Built-up handle spoons
	Sock aids
Bed rails—if confined to bed	Bath benches—certain types
	Dycem nonslip material

TABLE 3. COVERED AND NONCOVERED DURABLE MEDICAL EQUIPMENT (DME).

number in order to bill the DMERC for the DME. All occupational therapy practitioners who provide splints or other DMEPOS should apply for a supplier number (if they wish to supply and bill for the equipment themselves) or verify that the facility for whom they work has a supplier number through which Medicare can be billed. Practitioners in home health generally submit claims for DME provided to the patient through the agency or use a local medical supply dealer who will provide the equipment and submit the claim to the Medicare DMERC.

Certain items covered as DME may require a physician's order and a written rationale supporting the need for and use of the requested item. This is called a "Certificate of Medical Necessity." The occupational therapy practitioner may assist the physician and the DME provider by writing the rationale or offering information to support the rationale. After the paperwork is submitted, Medicare will review the request and determine the necessity and appropriateness. On items that require prior authorization, approval must be received before the equipment is ordered.

DME is reimbursed under Medicare Part B. In Part B, Medicare will pay for 80% of the allowable rental or purchase price of the equipment. Allowable cost is determined by Medicare. Many home health agencies do not choose to handle DME provisions through their own agency. If this is the case, the practitioner will need to refer the patient to a local DME dealer who can supply the equipment and bill Medicare Part B through the DMERC. Occupational therapists can also apply to Medicare to receive a supplier number as a DME dealer and may supply DME equipment to patients and bill Medicare Part B directly.

How then can the home health occupational therapy practitioner best assist his or her patients in getting the equipment that they need? The therapist's role moves into that of an educator and facilitator—educating the patient/family about the types of equipment needed and facilitating its acquisition by directing the patient to appropriate suppliers. Several strategies are suggested:

- Collect catalogs that offer equipment to show patients and distribute order forms.
- Survey your community and become aware of the retail medical suppliers and DME dealers.
- Survey your community for local organizations and clubs that may have various types of equipment such as commodes, wheelchairs, and toilet seats for loan or temporary use.
- Refer patient/family to appropriate resources.

When recommending the purchase of equipment, the practitioner needs to aware of what the family's and patient's financial obligations may be. If the equipment is approved DME and is payable under Part B, the patient/family will be responsible for 20% of the allowable cost. If the recommended equipment is not considered DME, the patient/family will be responsible for 100% of the cost.

E. Review of Service/Denial of Payment

Periodically during the treatment process, Medicare's designated intermediary (a financial and medical review body assigned to a specific region of the country) reviews the appropriateness of the frequency of visits, the date of onset, and the documented progress. The reviewers are generally nurses who may or may not be familiar with occupational therapy. Thus, the quality of visit-related documentation plays a very important role in obtaining reimbursement. Good documentation demonstrates the progress necessary for reimbursement, and it also serves as justification for continued treatment or the termination of care. Medicare intermediaries look for significant practical and functional improvement that is well-paced over a reasonable period. Denials of Medicare coverage occur when:

- Eligibility criteria are not met (e.g., patient is not homebound, lacks physician orders, and/or need for intermittent physical therapy, speech-language pathology, or skilled nursing on an intermittent basis is not evident);
- the need for occupational therapy's skilled service is not reasonable or necessary;
- significant progress has not been documented (See Chapter 8 on documentation);

- duplication of services exists; and/or
- fraud and abuse of program policies occurs.

Practitioners should realize that denial can always be appealed when a reasonable justification exists that is consistent with Medicare guidelines. Medicare provides for a formal appeals process that home health agencies may use. Practitioners are encouraged to pursue this process and participate when warranted. Check with your agency regarding the exact procedure. It is not uncommon for denials to be reversed when further information is presented and careful review of documentation is conducted.

III. Medicaid

Medicaid is a federally regulated, state-administered program. Its purpose is to provide health care to the poor and medically indigent. The cost of the program is shared by the state and federal government. The 1967 Social Security Amendments, which went into effect in 1970, require most states to provide home health coverage to Medicaid beneficiaries who are also eligible for care in a skilled nursing facility. Coverage varies from state to state because under Medicaid, occupational therapy is considered an optional service. Medicaid differs from Medicare in that the three qualifying skilled services (nursing, physical therapy, and speech-language pathology) are not necessarily prerequisites for occupational therapy and the patient may need not always be homebound (Trossman, 1984). However, this interpretation varies from state to state, so the regulation in a particular state should be checked.

Overall, limits on Medicaid reimbursement rates are significantly lower than Medicare, and increasing numbers of agencies are turning away Medicaid recipients. A few states allow therapists to receive individual Medicaid provider numbers. These therapists can accept assignments and bill Medicaid directly for occupational therapy in the home. Current eligibility for a Medicaid benefit period should be checked before services begin because prior authorization to start services can vary dramatically, slowing the initiation of treatment.

Home health agencies that wish to provide services to Medicaid recipients must demonstrate certification under Medicare before submitting any charges. Patients covered by both Medicare and Medicaid who receive home health services are expected to sign the appropriate forms so that the agency will submit claims to Medicare first and then file additional claims with Medicaid. Most Medicaid programs require that services be rendered in a patient's own residence or that of a relative, and that a plan of care be established by the patient's attending physician.

IV. Private Insurance

Benefits for occupational therapy under private health insurance plans vary greatly. Most basic hospital and major medical policies provide benefits for inpatient hospital occupational therapy services, but coverage for outpatient or home health services is less uniform. Generally, policies either specifically mention occupational therapy as a covered service or it is not specifically mentioned. Rarely is occupational therapy named as being excluded. However, when occupational therapy services are not specifically named, it is advisable to check with the insurer and explain the services to be offered. Often such action will result in appropriate coverage.

Private insurance plans are more likely than Medicare to place limits on frequency and the duration of therapy visits as well as the amount that will be paid. Some policies require a copayment from the insured to assist with costs.

It is important to remember that benefits are confirmed policy by policy. That is, two patients with the same insurance carrier and with levels of insurance benefits that appear to be similar, may indeed have different access to services. Because of this lack of consistency in coverage within and between companies, the type of benefits available are usually investigated by the home health agency before it accepts a referral.

V. Managed Care Plans

Managed care plans are an alternative to the traditional model of insurance service delivery. They were originally mandated by Congress in the 1970s and were designed to govern care in a way that would decrease costs. They have grown dramatically and a large proportion of the population is currently insured under some form of a managed care plan.

One of the most popular forms of managed care plans is the health maintenance organization (HMO). HMOs provide a comprehensive range of services to their members. Members pay a fixed premium at regular intervals and receive health care services that are needed without any additional costs or only a small copayment. To remain successful and retain their ability to attract and keep members, as well as remain profitable, HMOs must provide needed services to satisfy their members yet not over use services and threaten their prof-

itability. Most HMOs provide a basic home health benefit that covers the traditional Medicare home health services such as nursing and physical therapy. Occupational therapy may or may not be included in the HMO plans available in any one area. HMOs that serve Medicare beneficiaries (called federally qualified HMOs) must provide all of the benefits Medicare provides including occupational therapy. The need to produce a positive financial outcome will often dictate the decision regarding how many occupational therapy visits may be provided in any HMO plan. Practitioners can influence this decision by becoming aware of who makes the decision about the service delivery in the HMO and by clearly articulating the positive patient outcomes and resulting financial savings provided by occupational therapy interventions.

When occupational therapy is covered as a benefit, limitations on the number of home health visits are often set. Coordination among disciplines becomes important when the HMO limits total home health visits. Disciplines must decide the most advantageous way to divide services and achieve the best patient outcome.

The preferred provider organization (PPO) is another form of managed care that is a blend of a private pay plan and an HMO. It is an arrangement for service delivery. Members of a PPO pay a set premium but their choice of service providers, although broader than in an HMO, is more restricted than in a purely private pay plan and often an additional copayment for service is required. Service providers are designated as "preferred" and consist of groups or individuals with whom the PPO has negotiated set and agreed upon fees that are often discounted (Scott & Somers, 1992). "Nonpreferred" providers may be used by PPO members but the member will have to pay the higher proportion of the costs. A home health agency may be a designated provider in a PPO.

Most PPOs offer home health benefits. Provision of a home health benefit in a PPO varies. As with an HMO, preauthorization and limitations on the number of visits is very common when home health is covered by a PPO.

VI. The Veterans Administration

Although not a major reimbursement source for most home health agencies, the Veterans Administration (VA) reimburses providers for certain home health services if specific qualifying conditions are fulfilled. First, the patient must be homebound, and second, services must be ordered by a physician. The diagnosis to be treated may be either a service-related condition (e.g., diabetes that developed during the veteran's active duty and was treated at that time); or a nonservice-connected condition that has been reviewed by a rating board to determine the veteran's eligibility for the Aid and Attendance Homebound Program. Reimbursement from the VA is contingent on prior approval in the latter case, which is obtained from VA regional offices, and not directly from the VA hospital.

VII. The Civilian Health and Medical Program of the Uniformed Services (CHAMPUS)

Home health service as a designated benefit is not provided under the CHAMPUS program. However, occupational therapy is covered on both an inpatient and outpatient basis when provided by a CHAMPUS authorized institutional provider as part of an organized rehabilitation program (Office of the Civilian Health and Medical Program of the Uniformed Service, 1989). If outpatient occupational therapy services are provided in the patient's home but still billed by the CHAMPUS authorized institutional provider, the service can be covered. Since the majority of home health agencies are not authorized institutional providers, service delivery and billing are not usually done by these agencies. CHAMPUS does offer a Home Health Demonstration Program whereby a patient can receive service in the home if the cost is cheaper.

VIII. Federal Employees' Blue Cross/Blue Shield

The Federal Employees' Blue Cross/Blue Shield plan offers both a high option and a standard option to its members. The high option provides more extensive coverage than the standard option with a lower deductible and copayments for the insured. Occupational therapy is covered under both options on an outpatient basis, but is covered on a home health basis only under the high option plan. The occupational therapy that is provided must be part of an approved home health care program.

IX. Ethical Issues

As the demand for health care services has grown and reimbursement has become more available, the competition for the reimbursement dollar has increased. As a result, service providers have become more bottom-line sensitive, and reimbursement issues often assume a central role in decision making and planning. The pressures to "maximize" reimbursement are felt in all arenas of practice and appear to be intensifying. In the home health setting, these pressures can be problematical for the practitioner.

Practitioners in home health need to be sensitive to the reimbursement pressures that can influence their practice as well as be aware of the ethical and legal problems they may present. Fraud and abuse in reimbursement can occur in many ways, but perhaps the most common problems in home health are billing the insurer for treatment that was not actually provided; or providing very brief or minimal service while seeking full reimbursement. These practices can occur more easily in home health than in some other settings due to the isolated nature of home health service delivery. Therapy providers see patients alone and other agency representatives are not available to verify or check whether services were actually provided or how long they lasted. The fact that service providers may be working on a contractual basis that ties their own income into the number of visits they complete can provide a tempting opportunity for some practitioners to "pad" the number of visits they perform in order to increase their income. General productivity standards that target the expected number of visits employees are expected to complete can also pressure practitioners who may be behind in their work, to document treatment visits that may not have occurred.

Each of these situations presents the practitioner with an ethical decision. Individuals practicing in home health should be alert to the possible conflicting pressures and values they may experience and how to address them. Awareness of possible problems in this area can sensitize the practitioner to recognizing a problem when it occurs and assist them in personally avoiding fraudulent and abusive practices. Practitioners also need to be alert as to what is occurring around them. Each individual has a professional and ethical responsibility to report fraud and abuse when it is identified or observed. Efforts to bring the problem to the attention of the individuals involved and their supervisors should occur first. If the problems are not remedied, abuse should be reported to higher authorities. Medicare, for example, maintains a 24-Hour Fraud and Abuse Hotline (800-368-5779) that can be used to report violations.

X. Conclusion

It is important to emphasize that occupational therapy practitioners should confirm the guidelines for reimbursement for occupational therapy directly with their agency and/or third-party payer. Lack of coverage or denial of coverage should not be accepted as a final decision. Often additional contact with the third-party payer and further explanation of the services provided can change the initial decision.

Just as importantly, occupational therapy practitioners should keep abreast of legislative and regulatory changes that affect the practice of home health. Advocacy and participation in the political process are a necessary function of health care professionals in today's environment. Without an understanding of reimbursement guidelines and legislative or regulatory initiatives, occupational therapists and occupational therapy assistants will find it very difficult to provide quality care to patients. This is the profession's primary goal.

References

Health Care Financing Administration. (1990). *Medicare intermediary manual, Part 3, Claims process* (DHHS Transmittal No. 1487, Section 3906.4). Washington, DC: U.S. Government Printing Office.

Health Care Financing Administration. (1989). *Medicare home health agency manual.* (Publication No. HIM 11). Baltimore: Author.

Office of the Civilian Health and Medical Program of the Uniformed Service. (1989). *Champus policy manual.* (6010.47-M). Aurora, CO. Author.

Scott, S., & Somers, F. (1992). Payment for occupational therapy services. In J. Bair & M. Gray (Eds.), *The occupational therapy manager.* Rockville, MD: American Occupational Therapy Association.

Trossman, P. (1984). Administrative and professional issues for the occupational therapist in home health care. *American Journal of Occupational Therapy, 38*(11), 726–733.

Chapter 12

Employee and Independent Contractor Relationships With the Home Health Agency

Considerations for the Therapist

by Rebecca Austill-Clausen,
MS, OTR, FAOTA,

with contributions from
Michael J. Steinhauer,
OTR, MPH, FAOTA,
and Barry H. Frank, Esq.

I. Introduction

With the rapid growth of the home health industry, a variety of services have become available to homebound patients. Occupational therapy plays an important role in total rehabilitation, enabling individuals receiving services to obtain their maximum level of independence in the home. As more occupational therapy practitioners enter this treatment setting to practice, the profession and home health industry must develop a working relationship to meet each other's needs and still satisfy their own. This chapter highlights the responsibilities of occupational therapists, occupational therapy assistants, and home health agencies when entering into this relationship, and also defines types of agreements that may be negotiated at the beginning of therapy work relationships.

There may be situations that put occupational therapy practitioners, practicing as independent contractors, in conflict with Medicare regulations. It is suggested that occupational therapy practitioners discuss their specific job responsibilities with the home health agency and clarify the different parameters for occupational therapy practitioners practicing as independent contractors or identified as employees. It is important that each party have an appreciation and an understanding of the other's needs and limits, given the parameters of third-party reimbursement for agency costs and the regulations defining independent contractor relationships.

Home health agencies can provide occupational therapy services to their patients by hiring occupational therapy practitioners as full-time or part-time employees or they may hire occupational therapy practitioners who identify themselves as independent contractors. The latter method has become more common in recent years.

The use of occupational therapists and occupational therapy assistants as independent contractors has advantages for both home health agencies and the practitioner. For home health agencies, it is cost effective because there is no need to provide benefits, leave, equipment, or withhold taxes. Further, the home health agencies can expand or reduce staff to meet their needs without making an expensive commitment to full-time employees. Independent contractor practitioners maintain a high level of productivity, and the home health agency is reimbursed for their services by third-party payers at a rate that includes the individual's fee and the agency's overhead, up to a limit. Thus, the cost of providing occupational therapy is usually completely funded by third-party reimbursement.

For practitioners, working as an independent contractor can offer tremendous flexibility and independence. There are benefits particularly important to individuals interested in raising a family while maintaining a job, attending graduate school, or desiring more free time. Independent contractors should be responsible for their own scheduling, choosing their own hours, and determining where and when they want to treat their clients. In addition, the occupational therapy practitioner can benefit from all the other advantages of having their own private practice. These benefits may include such amenities as tax write-offs (a review of the most recent tax law is recommended), greater control over personal income, and independence from bureaucracy. Usually, independent contractors receive greater gross pay (hourly or visit rate) than employees because independent contractors are responsible for providing their own benefits, equipment, insurance, and tax withholdings.

When practitioners work as employees, the employer may provide health insurance, withhold taxes, provide vacation, sick and personal leave days, supply equipment and forms, and furnish liability and worker's compensation insurance, and possibly, a retirement plan.

II. Independent Contractor vs. Employee: Comparing Characteristics in Home Health

Table 1 describes the general difference between occupational therapy practitioners working as independent contractors or as employees for home health agencies. This information is presented only as a guideline. Occupational therapy practitioners are strongly advised to study the Internal Revenue Service parameters classifying workers as employees or independent contractors

Occupational therapy practitioners are also advised to obtain advice from a knowledgeable certified public accountant or tax attorney to help clarify the different conditions for practitioners working as employees or independent contractors (Austill-Clausen & Frank, 1994; Internal Revenue

Service Form SS-8, 1993; Revenue Proc., 1985; Revenue Rul., 1987; The Revenue Act of 1978).

Information in the next table is presented only as a guideline. Each home health agency may interpret this data differently, and occupational therapy practitioners are advised to consult with their respective agencies regarding the following parameters. Also, the employee guidelines listed are based on the assumption that the occupational therapy employee is reimbursed on an hourly basis, rather than on a per-visit basis.

III. Elements of Contracts

In forming relationships with home health agencies, full-time salaried employee practitioners should consider elements of professional security, just as independent contract practitioners do. Regardless of work status, occupational therapists and occupational therapy assistants should consider the following elements for inclusion in their contracts.

Generally, contracts need to define the occupational therapy practitioner's and the agency's respective responsibilities, and account for fees and charges. Contracts should serve as a formal means of communication between the parties.

A. Purpose
The purpose of a contract should be expressed in the following elements:
- A statement addressing why and how agencies provide services in the home and identifying the need for occupational therapy. Usually these statements begin, "Whereas...," and they are intended to create an understanding the of conditions that brought the service provider and the agency together.
- An accompanying statement about the compensation of occupational therapists and occupational therapy assistants as full-time hourly employees, or as independent contractors paid on a per-visit basis. Occupational therapy practitioners need to understand the reason a home health agency pays its therapists as employees or independent contractors so they are able to clarify their relationship with the home health agency.

B. General Responsibilities and Expectations of the Agency
The contract should state certain responsibilities that the agency will assume and certain expec-

tations that it may have of the practitioner. Consider the following:

- The agency's responsibility to receive referrals completely and accurately, to secure a physician's orders for care, to determine a patient's eligibility before his or her referral to occupational therapy, and to collect charges to pay its staff.
- If possible, some of the general guidelines such as visit parameters for third-party reimbursement of services, identifying also the

health profession involved (occupational therapy). Although the practice is not recommended, some contracts specify diagnostic groups and related "frequency and duration" guides not to be exceeded by field staff. Agencies include such specifications to gain a greater control of costs and potential denials.

- The agency's responsibility to provide orientation sessions and regularly scheduled clinical and administrative supervision for its employees. The home health agency also

Parameters	Independent Contractors	Employees
Contract	usually	not always
Per-visit reimbursement	usually	usually paid hourly
Mileage reimbursement	no	usually
Travel time reimbursement	no	yes
Equipment/supplies	no	yes
Paid consultation time	no	yes
Paid malpractice insurance	no	yes
Paid medical insurance	no	yes
Supervision/control	no	yes
Flexible schedule	yes	no
Right to refuse referrals	yes	no
Reimbursement for meetings	negotiable	yes
Reimbursement for no-show visits	negotiable	yes
Telephone call reimbursement	no	yes
Paid elective in-services	negotiable	yes
Paid documentation time	not usually	yes
Need to invoice agency	yes	no
Taxes withheld	no	yes
Paid workers' compensation	no	yes
Paid unemployment	no	yes
Tax Reporting Form 1099	yes	no
Tax Reporting Form W2	no	yes

TABLE 1. INDEPENDENT CONTRACTOR VS. EMPLOYEE PARAMETERS IN HOME HEALTH.

Table adapted from *Independent Contractor or Employee. How To Satisfy the IRS* by R. Austill-Clausen and B.H. Frank, 1994, Rockville, MD: American Occupational Therapy Association.

needs to define its organizational structure and clarify administrative (not supervisory) roles for therapists working as independent contractors, since independent contractors are not supervised or controlled, according to Internal Revenue Service regulations. (Austill-Clausen et al, 1994; Frank, 1989)

- The agency's responsibility to designate referrals for occupational therapy in terms of usual and customary referral call-in procedures and predetermined arrangements for time allotment. The agency should ensure complete and accurate information (to the best of its ability) and denote a timely sequence for initiating, accepting, and acting on referrals.

- The agency's responsibility to provide medical and personal liability coverage for their employees. Most agencies cover all of their field staff employee insurance needs automatically, but this should not be assumed. The level of malpractice insurance coverage should also be defined and made a part of the contract. This may hold for automobile insurance as well, because field staff spend much of their time in their vehicles. Premium payments for all insurance coverage should be clarified as part of the negotiated benefits. On the other hand, independent contractors are responsible for providing all of their own insurance needs.

- The agency's responsibility to provide assistance with scheduling and assignment particulars. The agency can make known its intent to keep the occupational therapy practitioner up-to-date on changes in address, scheduling preferences of the patient, physician assignments, and the medical condition of the patient. The contract may specify the intent of the agency to provide such assistance in this process and may define the frequency of and the mechanism for these communications.

- Rate of pay considerations (e.g., the rate of payment for services for visits and evaluations, travel allowances, consultation charges, fees for assuming supervisory responsibility, and costs of attending meetings). Regularly scheduled or previously agreed upon visits when the patient is not at home may be reimbursed at a reduced rate. Contracts vary greatly in all these areas and are primarily determined by local market factors at any given moment. Some

occupational therapists and occupational therapy assistants prefer to be paid weekly, some every other week, and some monthly. Others care less about the frequency of pay and more about the itemization of bills for services (i.e., the breakdown of their rate of pay into visit charges, travel charges, and meeting charges). However, full-time staff employees do not need to exercise such discipline; they adhere to their agency's general policy on reimbursement for such items. In any event, this section should be clearly defined, attempting to take into account all reasonable professional and visit-related expenses.

- Tax withholding will differ between employees and independent contractors. Employers traditionally withhold federal, state, and local taxes, social security, and worker's compensation. Independent contractors are responsible for withholding their own federal, state, and local taxes, unemployment, worker's compensation (if desired), and both the employer and employee components of the social security payment.

- The agency's policy with regard to recoupment of fees paid for visits that are later denied reimbursement. Most agency administrative staff do not hold an occupational therapist or an occupational therapy assistant responsible for denials, except in the event of a clearly uninformed judgment on documentation that results in an unappealable denial. For example, if an occupational therapy practitioner documents that the patient was "out driving" or "mowing the lawn" on the practitioner's arrival, the payer will probably deem the patient "not homebound" and deny the charges outright. An agency may then hold the occupational therapy practitioner responsible for a lack of insight in submitting medical justification. Agencies are, to a greater extent, including policies on denials as a part of their contracts with field staff.

- The agency's expectation for the therapist to supervise other team members and occupational therapy assistants. Agency personnel frequently include such items to demonstrate to certification boards their organizational and contractual coverage of this aspect of staffing. The frequency and the content of supervision should be clearly defined, especially for those working as independent contractors. Independent contractors cannot be supervised, according to the Internal Revenue Service. (Austill-Clausen et al, 1994; Frank, 1989)

- The agency's philosophy regarding treating patients privately, once the patients are discharged from the home health agency. The majority of agencies consider this to be a conflict of interest situation and do not allow occupational therapy practitioners to treat the same patient privately that they initially treated through the home health agency.

C. General Responsibilities of the Occupational Therapy Practitioner

Many aspects of a contract are responsibilities of both the agency and the occupational therapy practitioner. Yet some matters fall directly to the practitioner for contract satisfaction such as the following:

- Provision of timely referral taking, initiation of services, occupational therapy evaluations, treatment planning, and direct skilled services to patients whose treatment plan requires occupational therapy intervention. The practitioner must also adhere to the scope of the physician's signed orders for care. In addition, he or she accepts responsibility for instruction to the family and others, and for communication with the physician for regular updates on the patient's condition. A definition in the contract of the general skilled professional responsibilities of the occupational therapist and the occupational therapy assistant is necessary and should include broad responsibilities incurred during treatment.
- In-service training responsibilities and frequencies, case-conference participation, and other continuing, patient-related duties. Charges for these requirements may be billed separately rather than as part of visit charges.
- Provision of periodic medical documentation for all services provided. The method of documentation may be specified (e.g., dictated to the agency, typed, or handwritten), as well as the method for its incorporation into the medical record (e.g., hand-delivered to the agency, mailed, or sent by messenger).
- Provision of documentation that the practitioner meets the health requirements of the

agency and has the qualifications for the position, and submission of an appropriate license and certification for the personnel record. Personal liability (malpractice) insurance is often required. (The American Occupational Therapy Association, Inc. offers professional liability policies at a group rate through its private insurance agreements.)

- Agreement to adhere to the policies and procedures of the agency in all business and professional matters. The contract may also include a statement that communications issued by the agency on policy changes will be incorporated into the practices of the occupational therapist or the occupational therapy assistant.
- Submission of bills for services at an agreed upon frequency and in a form appropriate to the needs of both parties. The content should include the necessary information to clearly distinguish time devoted to the agency's business from that spent on the provision of service.
- The practitioner's intention not to attempt to collect fees from any other party but the agency. The contract may state that patients and third-party payers should not be billed separately or directly for services that the agency should pay directly to the practitioner.
- Equipment ordering and treatment supplies in stock. It may be helpful as a rule, and appropriate as an interest of the practitioner, for the contract to include a statement about responsibility for equipment and supplies. Some agencies insist that the individual contractor in private practice maintain his or her own supply of demonstration equipment, whereas others prefer that the supply be based at and paid for by the agency, therefore making it available to all staff at the agency offices.
- Retention of all medical and business records for the appropriate and legal period, in the event that an agency audit requires books and records of contract staff. The retention of books and records is required by law, and the length of time that they must be retained varies from state to state.
- Clarification of tax paying procedures (taxes deducted per check for employees, or taxable compensation reported on Form 1099 at the year's end for independent contractors), and contract review periods. This

responsibility is shared by the practitioner and the agency.

D. General Provisions

As a rule, all contracts reflect the following:

- The length of the contract, with the beginning date and provision for periodic review and renegotiation (usually annually). In order for the home health agency to receive Medicare reimbursement, an annual performance evaluation of the practitioner is required, and usually accompanies the contract renewal. Copies of the contract and performance evaluation are to be made available on request.
- A job description, initialed by both parties, with periodic review. The job description is often different for therapists working as a staff employee or as an independent contractor. The employee job description usually includes control and supervision variables, while the independent contractor job description does not have such specificity.
- A statement about the confidentiality of the contract and the patient's records.
- A statement concerning "assignability" for satisfaction of the contract. For instance, if one occupational therapist desires to hire another to go on visits or cover the in-service training aspect of the contract, a question may arise about the legitimacy of the substitution and the contracting occupational therapy practitioner's right to do so. In the event that a practitioner desires such an extended agreement, a clause to this effect should be added.

It is strongly recommended that the occupational therapy practitioner review the completed contract with an attorney before he or she signs it.

E. Reimbursement Parameters

1. Home Health Agency

Under the Medicare program, home health agencies are reimbursed on the basis of their actual costs up to an aggregate cost limit. These limits are updated annually by the Health Care Financing Administration (HCFA) and make distinctions for whether an agency is located in an urban or rural area, and for salary differences among areas.

Briefly, cost limits are computed for each type of service (i.e., nursing, occupational therapy, physical therapy, speech-language pathology, social work, aide) provided by home health agencies. When a home health agency files its annual cost report, a form that calculates an aggregate limit (the sum of each discipline's per-visit limit multiplied by the actual number of visits performed in that discipline) is included. This total cost limit is compared to the agency's total cost (the sum of each discipline's actual cost). Medicare reimburses the lower of the costs or the aggregate limit.

Charges for each discipline, including occupational therapy, are used by Medicare as the basis for "interim payments" throughout the agency's fiscal year. Charges are established by estimating expected costs and utilization in a service, usually based on the previous year's visits and costs. Ultimately, the agency will receive its actual costs by Medicare up to the cost limit amount.

2. Independent Contractors

Charges billed to home health agencies by independent contractors appear on the cost report as part of the agency's costs. Medicare intermediaries must ensure that the costs of occupational therapy and other services provided by contractors and claimed by home health agencies are "reasonable" in accordance with regulations. In making "reasonable cost" determinations, intermediaries often employ the "prudent buyer" concept, which states that a provider's costs for any service may not exceed those costs that a prudent and cost-conscious buyer would incur based on market forces in a specific geographic area. Therefore, an independent contractor should ensure that their charges are not out of line with other practitioners, since a home health agency will be reluctant to pay a charge in excess of what the Medicare intermediary may consider reasonable in the area.

Since 1983, Medicare has had the authority to implement salary equivalency guidelines for occupational therapy services under arrangements such as those that are contractual. As of November 1994, rates had been established only for physical therapy and respiratory therapy. Unless HCFA subsequently publishes a Federal Register notice instituting rates for occupational therapy services, the policy reflected above will remain (HCFA, 1983).

3. Occupational Therapy Assistant

Occupational therapy assistants who, by applicable state occupational therapy regulations (where they exist), and who work under the supervision of occupational therapists, are generally reimbursed for visits at a lower rate than their supervisors. However, the agency's charge to the third-party payer is usually the same for visits by either category of personnel. When joint visits by the occupational therapist and the occupational therapy assistant are made for supervisory or other purposes, fee splitting is appropriate and encouraged. The two practitioners involved may prearrange to share the one fee charged to the agency.

F. Group Practice Arrangements

A growing number of occupational therapy practitioners are forming professional groups to offer practitioners' services to home health agencies. Generally an officer of the group or the corporation takes responsibility for signing contracts with agencies and facilitates service delivery at specific home health agencies. Factors noted earlier for inclusion in a contract between an individual and an agency should be included in this group agency arrangement. An additional clause providing for substitution of therapists should be present in the agreement.

IV. Conclusion

The practice of occupational therapy in the home is an exciting and challenging area for independent-minded occupational therapy practitioners. A variety of aspects and considerations not customarily associated with the provision of health care in other settings are featured. Occupational therapists and occupational therapy assistants are encouraged to carefully expand their practice in this new and growing field. With a working knowledge of reimbursement provisions, clinical delivery mechanisms, professional and legal guidelines, and the personal attributes necessary for success, occupational therapy practitioners will be able to contribute to a dynamic and successful component of this important area of practice.

References

Austill-Clausen, R., & Frank, B. (1994). *Independent contractor or employee. How to satisfy the IRS*. Rockville, MD: American Occupational Therapy Association.

Frank, B. (1989). Independent contractor vs. employee: Guidelines for the practitioner. In *The Practical Accountant*. New York: Warren, Gorham and Lamont.

Health Care Financing Administration. (1983). *Medicare-provided reimbursement manual* (Pub. 15), Section 2103. Washington, DC: U.S. Government Printing Office.

Internal Revenue Service Form SS-8, Determination of employee work status for purposes of federal employment taxes and income tax withholding (Revised July 1993; Expires 1996).

The Revenue Act of 1978, P.L. No.95–600, Section 530 (1978).

Revenue Proc. 85-18, C.B. 518 (1985-1).

Revenue Rul. 87-41, C.B. 296 (1987-1).

Appendixes

Appendix A

Basic Statistics About Home Care 1994

Reprinted with permission

BASIC STATISTICS
ABOUT HOME CARE 1994

National Association for Home Care
519 C Street, NE
Washington, DC 20002-5809

Contact: Val J. Halamandaris
202/547-7424
FAX: 202/547-3540

Home care in the United States is a diverse and rapidly growing service industry. About 15,000 providers deliver home care services to some 7 million individuals who require such services because of acute illness, long-term health conditions, permanent disability or terminal illness. Annual expenditures for home care are expected to exceed $23 billion in 1994.

1. Home Care Providers

The first home care agencies were established in the 1880s. Their numbers grew to some 1,100 by 1963 and to over 15,000 currently. Home health agencies, home care aide organizations, and hospices are known collectively as "home care agencies."

The National Association for Home Care (NAHC) has identified a total of 15,027 home care agencies in the US as of March 1994 (see Figure 1). This number consists of 7,521 Medicare-certified home health agencies, 1,459 Medicare-certified hospices, and 6,047 home health agencies, home care aide organizations, and hospices that do not participate in Medicare.

Figure 1. Home Care Agencies: Certified Home Health Agencies, Certified Hospices, and Others, 1989–1994

| Year | Total | Certified Agencies | | |
		HHAs	Hospices	Other
1989	11,097	5,676	597	4,824
1990	11,765	5,695	774	5,296
1991	12,433	5,780	898	5,755
1992	12,497	6,004	1,039	5,454
1993	13,959	6,497	1,223	6,239
1994	15,027	7,521	1,459	6,047

Source: NAHC inventory of home care agencies.

a. Medicare-Certified Agencies

Home care agencies of various types have been providing high-quality, in-home services to Americans for over a century. However, Medicare's enactment in 1965 greatly accelerated the industry's growth. Medicare made home health services, primarily skilled nursing and therapy of a curative or restorative nature, available to the elderly and, beginning in 1973, to certain disabled younger Americans.

Between 1967 and 1980, the number of agencies certified to participate in the Medicare program nearly doubled, from 1,753 to 2,924. Between 1980 and 1985, the number of agencies nearly doubled again to 5,983.

In the mid-1980s, the number of Medicare-certified home health agencies leveled off at around 5,900 as a result of increasing Medicare paperwork and unreliable payment policies. These problems led to a lawsuit brought against the Health Care Financing Administration in 1987 by a coalition of US Congressmembers led by Reps. Harley Staggers (D-WV) and Claude Pepper (D-FL), consumer groups, and NAHC. The successful conclusion of this lawsuit gave NAHC the opportunity to participate in a rewrite of the Medicare home health payment policies.

Since these revisions, Medicare's annual home health benefit outlays have increased significantly and the number of home health agencies has risen to an all-time high of 7,521 as of May 1994.

Hospital-based and proprietary agencies have grown faster than any other type of certified agency since the coverage clarifications. Proprietary agencies now comprise more than a third, and hospital-based agencies equal nearly a third of all certified agencies. This differs markedly from the industry composition in the early 1980s, when public health agencies dominated the ranks of certified agencies and proprietary and hospital-based agencies combined accounted for only one-fourth of the total. Figure 2 on the next page shows the changes in the types of agencies participating in Medicare.

Figure 2. Number of Medicare-Certified Home Health Agencies, by Auspice, 1967-1994

Year	Freestanding HHAs						Facility Based HHAs			
	VNA	COMB	PUB	PROP	PNP	OTH	HOSP	REHAB	SNF	TOTAL
1967	549	93	939	0	0	39	133	0	0	1,753
1975	525	46	1,228	47	0	109	273	9	5	2,242
1980	515	63	1,260	186	484	40	359	8	9	2,924
1985	514	59	1,205	1,943	832	4	1,277	20	129	5,983
1986	510	62	1,192	1,915	826	4	1,341	17	117	5,984
1987	500	61	1,172	1,882	803	1	1,382	14	108	5,923
1988	496	55	1,073	1,846	766	1	1,439	12	97	5,785
1989	491	51	1,011	1,818	727	1	1,465	10	102	5,676
1990	474	47	985	1,884	710	0	1,486	8	101	5,695
1991	476	41	941	1,970	701	0	1,537	9	105	5,780
1992	530	52	1,083	1,962	637	28	1,623	3	86	6,004
1993	594	46	1,196	2,146	558	41	1,809	1	106	6,497
5/94	586	45	1,146	2,892	597	48	2,081	3	123	7,521

Source: HCFA, Office of Survey and Certification.

VNA: Visiting Nurse Associations are freestanding, voluntary, non-profit organizations governed by a board of directors and usually financed by tax-deductible contributions as well as by earnings.

COMB: Combination agencies are combined government and voluntary agencies. These agencies are sometimes included with counts for VNAs.

PUB: Public agencies are government agencies operated by a state, county, city, or other unit of local government having a major responsibility for preventing disease and for community health education.

PROP: Proprietary agencies are freestanding, for-profit home health agencies.

PNP: Private not-for-profit agencies are freestanding and privately developed, governed, and owned nonprofit home health agencies.

OTH: Other freestanding agencies are agencies that do not fit one of the categories for freestanding agencies listed above.

HOSP: Hospital-based agencies are operating units or departments of a hospital. Agencies that have working arrangements with a hospital, or perhaps are even owned by a hospital but operated as separate entities, are classified as freestanding agencies under one of the categories listed above.

REHAB: Refers to agencies based in rehabilitation facilities.

SNF: Refers to agencies based in skilled nursing facilities.

b. Certified Hospices

Medicare added hospice benefits in October 1983, ten years after the first hospice was established in the US. Hospices provide palliative medical care and supportive social, emotional, and spiritual services to the terminally ill and their families. The number of Medicare-certified hospices has grown from 31 in January 1984 to 1,459 in January 1994. (For a separate fact sheet giving detailed information on hospices, please contact the Hospice Association of America, 202/546-4759.)

c. Noncertified Agencies

The 6,047 noncertified home health agencies, home care aide organizations, and hospices that remain outside Medicare do so for a variety of reasons. Some do not provide the kinds of services that Medicare covers. For example, home care aide organizations that do not provide skilled nursing care are not eligible to participate in Medicare. About 20% of these noncertified agencies are involved primarily in the provision of homemaker-home health aide services; about 20% are primarily providing hospice and/or bereavement services; and about 13% are primarily providing high tech services. Most of the rest of these agencies offer a multiplicity of services.

2. Home Care Expenditures and Utilization

a. National

National expenditures for personal health care will total nearly $900 billion in 1994 . Of this amount, nearly two-thirds goes for hospital care and physicians' services. Home care expenditures comprise only a small fraction of national health spending.

Total home care spending is difficult to estimate. In annual estimates of national health care spending from both the Department of Health and Human Services and the Congressional Budget Office, home care spending is only partially identified. Neither of these sources includes the home care delivered by noncertified home care agencies or hospital-based home health agencies. The most comprehensive estimate of national home care spending comes from the National Medical Expenditures Survey (NMES), which is conducted every ten years by the Agency for Health Care Policy and Research. According to the 1987 NMES, $11.6 billion was spent on home care in that year[1]. To estimate current spending, this figure may be updated with information from FIND/SVP, a New York City market research firm, which estimates that the home care market grew at an annual rate of 10% between 1986 and 1991 and that it will grow at an annual rate of 12% from 1991 to 1996[2]. Using these estimates, total home care spending could be estimated at $23.7 billion in 1994. A separate study published this year by Lewin-VHI updated the 1987 NMES information to 1992 levels for an estimated $22.8 billion in total spending[3]. The Lewin estimates indicate an average annual growth rate of 14.6%, which if updated to 1994 would total $29.9 billion. Using either method, home care accounts for roughly 3% of national health care spending (see Figure 3).

Figure 3. National Health Care Expenditures, 1994

	Percent
Total personal health care	100 %
Hospital care	42
Physicians' services	21
Nursing home care	9
Drugs and other medical nondurables	9
Other professional services	6
Dentists' services	5
Home care*	3
Other personal health care	2
Vision products and other medical durables	2

Source: Office of National Health Statistics, revised to reflect estimates of total home care spending.
*Home care estimates reflect the $23.7 billion estimate derived from 1987 NMES data updated by FIND/SVP growth estimates. Numbers may not add due to rounding.

Medicare is the largest single payor of home care services. In 1992, Medicare spending accounted for more than a third of total home care expenditures. Other public funding sources for home care include Medicaid, the Older Americans Act, Title XX Social Services Block Grants, the Veteran's Administration, and CHAMPUS. Private insurance comprises only a small proportion of home care payments. Most home care services are financed through out-of-pocket payments (see Figure 4).

Figure 4. Sources of Payment for Home Care, 1992

Source of Payment	1992
Total	100.0%
Medicare	37.8
Medicaid	24.7
Private insurance	5.5
Out-of-pocket	31.4
Other	0.6

Source: NMES 1987 data and Lewin-VHI analysis for 1992.

NMES also gathered information on the average cost of home care visits. These figures can be updated using the Medicare rates of growth in per-visit charges. Figure 5 shows that the average home care visit cost $49 in 1987 and $66 in 1993.

Figure 5. Average Expense Per Home Care Visit

	1987	1994**
Average	$49	$70
Nurse	62	89
Therapist	57	82
Home health aide	34	49
Homemaker	33	47
Other*	56	80

Source: Altman B., Walden D. Home Health Care: Use, Expenditures and Sources of Payment. National Medical Expenditures Survey Research Findings 15. (AHCPR Pub. No. 93-0040) Agency for Health Care Policy and Research. Rockville, MD: Public Health Service.
*Includes social workers and other professionals.
**Updated by average annual rate of increase of Medicare per-visit charges: 5.3% between 1987 and 1992.

b. Medicare

The home health benefit represents a relatively small proportion of Medicare spending, only about 8% of total benefit payments in 1994 (see Figure 6). Over half of the estimated $167 billion Medicare benefit payments go to hospitals and nearly a quarter to physicians. Hospice payments account for less than 1% of total Medicare benefit payments.

Figure 6. Medicare Benefit Payments, 1994 (in millions)

	Amount	Percent
Total Medicare Benefit Payments*	$166,612	100.0 %
Total Part A	$105,924	63.6 %
Hospital care	84,614	50.8
Skilled nursing facility	6,334	3.8
Home health agency	13,787	8.3
Hospice	1,189	0.7
Total Part B	$60,688	36.4 %
Physician	37,712	22.6
Outpatient facilities	14,242	8.5
Home health agency	127	0.1
Group practice prepayment	6,084	3.7
Independent laboratory	2,524	1.5

Source: HCFA, Office of the Actuary, unpublished information used for FY94 Board of Trustees Report.
*Excludes peer review organization expenditures.

In 1994, 37 million aged and disabled persons will be enrolled in the Medicare program. About 3.3 million enrollees will receive home health services, which is nearly double the number of home health recipients in 1990. In the same period, Medicare home health expenditures have more than tripled from $3.9 billion in 1990 to an estimated $13.8 billion in 1994. Most of the new spending has occurred as a result of new visits, which increased from 69.6 million in 1990 to an estimated 218.6 million in 1994.

Growth in the Medicare home health benefit can be attributed to specific legislative expansions of the benefit and to a number of socio-demographic trends, which have fostered growth in the program from the beginning and which will no doubt continue to do so for many years to come. Figure 7 shows the growth over time in the Medicare home health benefit.

Medicare hospice expenditures have grown from $112 million in 1987 to an estimated $1.2 billion in 1994. If current trends continue, an estimated 308,219 beneficiaries will receive hospice services under Medicare in 1994. (More detailed information is in the hospice fact sheet.)

Figure 7. Medicare Home Health Expenditures, Clients, and Visits for Selected Years, 1967-1994

Year	Expenditures (millions)	Clients (1000s)	Visits (1000s)
1967	$46	n/a	n/a
1975	208	500	10,800
1980	662	957	22,428
1985	1,773	1,589	39,742
1986	1,796	1,600	38,359
1987	1,879	1,565	35,591
1988	2,033	1,582	37,154
1989	2,527	1,685	46,275
1990	3,864	1,940	69,569
1991	5,620	2,223	100,015
1992	7,878	2,565	135,012
1993	10,961	2,975	177,475
1994	13,787	3,345	218,595

Source: HCFA, Office of the Actuary, unpublished information prepared for FY94 Trustees Report.

c. Medicaid

As in the case of Medicare, home health services represent a relatively small part of total Medicaid payments. Figure 8 shows that of the 102 billion in Medicaid benefit payments, over half went for hospital and skilled nursing facility services. Home health services comprised about 5.5% of the payments. Hospice is an optional Medicaid service, which is currently offered by 36 states. Payments for hospice services are estimated at $129 million in FY93.

Figure 8. Medicaid Expenditures, by Type of Service, FY93

	Amount (millions)	Pct.
Total Vendor Payments (a)	$101,707	100.0%
Inpatient hospital	27,895	27.4
Nursing home (b)	25,431	25.0
Physician	6,952	6.8
Outpatient hospital	6,215	6.1
Home health	5,611	5.5
Hospice (c)	129	0.1
Prescription drugs	7,970	7.8

Source: HCFA, Division of Medicaid Statistics. Data are from the HCFA-2082 Form, with the exception of hospice data, which come from the HCFA-64 Form.
Note: (a) Total expenditures include hospice expenditures from the HCFA-64 Form plus payments for all service types included in HCFA-2082 Form, not just the eight service types listed. (b) Includes other intermediate care facility payments. (c) Hospice expenditures come from HCFA-64 Form. All other expenditures come from the HCFA-2082.

Figure 9 shows the growth in the Medicaid home health benefit since FY75. Between FY92 and FY93, expenditures increased from $4.8 billion to $5.6 billion, an increase of nearly 17%. It should be noted that these amounts do not reflect total home care spending under Medicaid. Missing is information not run through the Medicaid Statistical Information System (MSIS). When included, the total Medicaid spending for home health equals $6.8 billion for FY93. Nearly all of this amount (about 80%) goes for servcies provided through the optional home care and waiver programs.

Figure 9. Medicaid Home Health Expenditures, Clients, and Visits, for Selected Years, 1975-1993

Fiscal Year	Vendor Payments (millions)	Clients (1000s)	Visits (1000s)
1975	$70	343	n/a
1980	332	392	n/a
1985	1,120	535	n/a
1990	3,404	719	n/a
1991	4,101	812	70,601
1992	4,888	926	109,293
1993	5,601	1,067	109,078

Source: HCFA, Division of Medicaid Statistics. Data are derived from the HCFA-2802 form, which began collecting information on visits in FY91.

3. Home Care Recipients

Estimates indicate that as many as 9 to 11 million Americans need home care services[4]. Most will receive services from so-called informal caregivers—family members, friends, or others who provide uncompensated care. Some will also receive formal services (i.e., purchased or compensated services from home care providers).

The NMES findings indicate that 5.9 million individuals, roughly 2.5% of the US population, received formal home care services in 1987 (see Figure 10). Of these recipients, about half were over the age of 65, and the amount of home care they used tended to increase with age. About 40% of the home care recipients had functional limitations in one or more activities of daily living. Age and functional disability are likely predictors of the need for home care services.

A more recent survey, conducted by the National Center for Health Statistics, gathered valuable information on client diagnoses[5]. Figure 11 (see next page) shows that more than 25% of home care patients admitted to home health agencies in 1992 had conditions related to diseases of the circulatory system. Persons with heart disease, including congestive heart failure, made up 49% of all conditions in this group. Stroke, diabetes, and hypertension were also frequent admission diagnoses for home care patients.

Figure 10. National Home Care Usage, by Client Age and Functional Status, 1987

Characteristics	US Population (thousands)	Home Care Recipients		Average No. of Visits Per Recipient
		Number (thousands)	Percent of US Population	
Age in years				
All Ages	239,393	5,878	2.5%	44.0
Under 65	212,872	2,912	1.4	24.4
Under 6	24,838	621	2.5	4.3
6-17	41,950	251	0.6	14.9
18-39	86,340	863	1.0	22.8
40-64	59,744	1,183	2.0	37.9
65 and older	26,521	2,966	11.2	63.3
65-74	16,378	1,165	7.1	55.7
75-84	8,111	1,173	14.5	66.9
85 and Older	2,032	628	30.9	70.6
Functional Status				
No ADL/IADL difficulties	227,004	2,765	1.2	12.8
1 ADL difficulty only	4,910	871	17.7	43.4
1-2 ADL difficulties	4,625	1,060	22.9	61.0
3 or more ADL difficulties	2,854	1,183	41.4	102.0

Source: National Medical Expenditures Survey, 1987.

Figure 11. Percent of Current Clients Receiving Home Health and Hospice Care, by First-listed Diagnosis at Admission, 1992 – Preliminary Data

IDC-9-CM* Procedure Category	ICD-9-CM Code	Home Health percent	Hospice percent
All Current Clients		100.0%	100.0%
Infectious and parasitic diseases	001-139	1.7	4.2
Neoplasms	140-239	6.4	65.9
Endocrine, nutritional, and metabolic diseases, and immunity disorders	240-279	9.8	n/a
Diseases of the blood and blood forming organs	280-289	2.9	n/a
Mental Disorders	290-319	3.1	n/a
Diseases of the nervous system and sense organs	320-389	6.2	2.8
Diseases of the circulatory system	390-459	25.6	12.5
Diseases of the respiratory system	460-519	6.5	n/a
Diseases of the digestive system	520-579	3.5	n/a
Diseases of the genitourinary system	580-629	2.2	n/a
Complications of pregnancy, childbirth, and the pueperium	630-676	0.2	n/a
Diseases of the skin and subcutaneous tissue	680-709	4.6	n/a
Diseases of the musculoskeletal system and connective tissue	710-739	9.3	n/a
Congenital anomolies	740-759	0.7	n/a
Certain conditions originating in the perinatal period	760-779	0.8	n/a
Symptoms, signs, and ill-defined conditions	780-799	5.0	n/a
Injury and poisoning	800-999	7.3	n/a
All other or unknown		4.2	n/a

Source: NCHS Sample Survey, 1992.
*ICD-9-CM is International Classification of Diseases, Clinical Modification, Ninth Revision.
Figures may not add due to rounding.

Many hospital patients are discharged to home care services for continued rehabilitative care. As hospital stays shortened in the early 1980s, the percentage of Medicare patients discharged to home health care increased from 9.1% in 1981 to 17.9% in 1985, according to a study by Abt Associates. Figure 12 shows the five DRGs (diagnosis-related groups) most likely to result in home health utilization.

Figure 12. Percent of Medicare Hospital Patients Discharged to Home Health Care, 1985

DRG #	Description	Pct. Discharged to Home Care
14	Stroke	27.0%
88	COPD	17.7
127	Heart failure	20.3
209	Major joint procedures	34.3
210	Hip/femur procedures	34.6

Source: "Medicare Patients and Postacute Care: Who Goes Where?" Rand Corporation, November, 1989.

4. Caregivers

a. Informal Caregivers

Estimates indicate that almost three-quarters of severely disabled elders receiving home care services in 1989 relied solely on family members or other unpaid help. Eight of 10 informal caregivers provide unpaid assistance an average of four hours a day, seven days a week. Three quarters of informal caregivers are female, and nearly a third are over the age of 65[6].

b. Formal Caregivers

Formal caregivers include those professionals and paraprofessionals who provide in-home health care and personal care services. Little information is available on the total number of formal caregivers. Neither the Bureau of Labor Statistics nor the major organizations that collect information

Figure 13. Number of Home Care Workers, 1994

Type of Employee	Number of Employees	Employees per Agency
RNs	254,643	16.9
LPNs	34,757	2.3
Physical Therapists	48,460	3.2
Home Care Aides	171,346	11.4
Other	148,854	9.9
Totals	657,622	43.8

Source: NAHC estimates based on data from HCFA and BLS.

on health care providers gather detailed information on the entire home care industry. However, when combined with information on Medicare-certified agencies that is collected by the Health Care Financing Administration, a reasonable estimate of employees can be achieved. Figure 13 (see previous page) shows that the number of home care workers in home care agencies totaled 657,622 in 1994. On average, these employees worked 27.8 hours per week.

Home care agencies frequently ask for information on employee productivity. Several studies of nursing productivity reveal that nurses deliver an average of five visits per day (see Figure 14). Nurses who specialize in pediatric care average only 2.4 visits per day but IV nurses average as many visits as other nurses.

c. Compensation

NAHC conducts a survey each year, which collects information on the salary and benefits provided to four home health agency management positions and seven caregiver positions. The level of compensation paid to home health agency executives tends to vary according to the auspice of the employing agency, whereas the level of compensation paid to home health agency field staff tends to vary more by the geographic location of the employing agency than the agency's auspice. Summary results are provided in Figures 15 and 16.

Figure 14. Comparative Findings of Home Care Nurse Productivity

Study	Patients Per Day
1. Spoelstra, 1988	5.0
2. Caie-Lawrence, 1990	5.0
3. C.S. Hedtke, 1992:	4.8
a. Pediatric RNs	2.4
b. IV RNs	4.9

Sources:
1. Spoelstra S. Productivity of Registered Nurses in Home Health Care: a Nationwide Survey. *CARING Magazine*. 1988; 2(2):57-58.
2. Caie-Lawrence J. A. Time Study of Home Care Nurses Poster Presentation, Sixth National Nursing Symposium-Home Health Care. May 17, 1990; Ann Arbor, Mich.
3. Hedtke C. S. How do home care nurses spend their time? *Journal of Nursing Administrators*.1992; 22(1):18-22.

Figure 15. Average Compensation of Home Health Agency Executives, July 1993

Chief executive officer	$64,570
Chief operating officers	61,830
Chief financial officers	52,794
Directors of nursing	46,986

Source: Home Health Agency Compsensation Survey Report, Washington, DC: NAHC,1993.
Note: Compensation includes fringe benefit.

Figure 16. Average Compensation of Home Health Agency Caregivers as of July 1993

Caregiver	Salaried Minimum	Salaried Average	Per Visit Minimum	Per Visit Average	Per Hour Minimum	Per Hour Average
RNs	$31,022	$38,723	$25.83	$33.79	$14.31	$18.21
LPNs	21,792	27,040	18.54	21.53	10.07	12.69
PTs	39,962	50,495	39.51	44.86	19.93	24.82
OTs	35,840	45,890	39.78	43.66	18.44	23.23
STs	36,402	46,287	40.73	44.25	20.00	24.34
MSWs	29,797	36,781	40.38	45.44	15.15	19.08
HCAs	15,195	18,721	11.70	13.52	6.52	8.55

Source: Home Health Agency Compensation, Survey Report, Washington, DC: NAHC; 1993.
Note: Compensation does not include fringe benefits.

Endnotes:
1. Altman B., Walden D. *Home Health Care: Use, Expenditures and Sources of Payment* (AHCPR Pub. No. 93-0040). National Medical Expenditure Survey Research Findings 15, Agency for Health Care Policy and Research. Rockville, MD: Public Health Service; 1993.
2. *The Market for Home Care Services*. New York, NY: FIND/SVP, Inc.; 1992.
3. Lewin-VHI anaylsis of NMES data. *The Heavy Burden of Home Care*. Washington, DC: Families USA; 1993.
4. US Bipartisan Commission on Comprehensive Health Care. *The Pepper Commission Final Report: A Call for Action*. Washington, DC: US Government Printing Office; 1990. S. Prt.101-114.
5. Strahan G. Overview of Home Health and Hospice Care Patients: Preliminary Data from the 1992 National Home and Hospice Care Survey. Advance data from vital and health statistics; no 235. Hyattsville, MD: National Center for Health Statistics; 1993.
6. *Pepper Commission Final Report*.

5. Cost-effective Home Care

In many cases, home care is a cost-effective service, not only for individuals recuperating from a hospital stay but also for those who, because of a functional or cognitive disability, are unable to take care of themselves. The following section lists some examples of cost-effective home care. However, it should be noted that cost-effectiveness is not the only rationale for home care. In fact, the best argument for home care may be that it is a humane and compassionate way to deliver health care and supportive services. Home care reinforces and supplements the care provided by family members and friends and maintains the recipient's dignity and independence, qualities that are all too often lost in even the best institutions.

Figure 17. Comparison of Hospital, SNF and Home Health Charges, 1991 and 1993 estimate

	1992	1994*
Hospital Charges Per Day	$1,459	$1,756
Skilled Nursing Facility Charges Per Day	264	284
Home Health Charges Per Visit	75	83

Source: Hospital and SNF Data are from Social Security Bulletin, Annual Statistical Supplemental 1993; Home Health information is from HCFA/BDMS.
*Estimate based on CPI index for various medical care items.

Figure 18. Cost of Inpatient Care Compared to Home Care, Selected Conditions

Conditions	Per Month Hospital Costs	Per Month Home Care Costs	Per Month Dollar Savings
a. Low birth weight	$26,190	$330	$25,860
b. Ventilator dependent adults	21,570	7,050	14,520
c. Oxygen dependent children	12,090	5,250	6,810

Source: (a) Casiro, O.G., McKenzie, M.E., McFayden, L, Shapiro, C., Seshia, M.M.K., MacDonald, N., Moffat, M, & Cheang, M.S., (1993). Earlier discharge with community-based intervention for low birth rate infants: a randomized trial. *Pediatrics*, 92(1), 128-134.

(b) Bach, J.R., Intinola, P., Alba, A.S., & Holland, I.E., (1992). The ventilator-assisted individual: cost analysis of institutionalization vs. rehabilitation and in-home management. *Chest*, 101(1), 26-30.

(c) Fields, A.I., Rosenblatt, A., Pollack, M.M., & Kaufman, J. (1991). Home care cost-effectiveness for respiratory technology-dependent children. *American Journal of Diseases of Children*, 145, 729-733.

Several research studies conducted in the past several years have compared inpatient care to home care costs for a specific group of patients. The cost savings data for three of these studies is summarized in Figure 18. The information has been aggregated at a monthly level for purposes of comparison.

Several additional studies of home care cost-effectiveness are summarized in the following paragraphs.

a. Psychiatric Care

An in-home crisis intervention program developed for psychiatric patients in Connecticut was effective in reducing hospital admissions, length of stay and readmissions. A two-year analysis of more than 600 patients showed that 80.7% of patients referred for hospital care could be treated at home instead. When inpatient admissions were necessary, the average length of stay could be reduced from 11.97 days to 7.48 days by adding elements of the in-home care program; and patients who received home care services were less likely to be readmitted for hospital care (11.8% of home care patients were readmitted compared to 45.9% of patients who did not receive home care services). (Source: Pigott, H.E., & Trott, L. (1993). Translating research into practice; the implementation of an in-home crisis intervention triage and treatment service in the private sector. *American Journal of Medical Quality*, 8(3), 138-144.

b. Terminally Ill Veterans

A home care program for terminally veterans reduced hospital per-capita costs by $971. In the six-month study, patients receiving home care used 5.9 fewer hospital days than those in the control group. No differences were found in patient survival, activities of daily living, cognitive functioning, or morale. However, patient and caregiver satisfaction with care was significantly better among the patients receiving home care. (Source: Hughes, S.L., Cummings, J., Weaver, F., Manheim, L. Braun, B., & Conrad, K. (1992). A randomized trial of the cost effectiveness of VA hospital-based home care for the terminally ill. *Health Services Research*, 26(6), 801-817.

c. Patients with COPD

An innovative home care program for patients with chronic obstructive pulmonary disease (COPD) that was tested in Connecticut found significant cost savings. The overall goal of the program was to provide more comprehensive home care servcies to COPD patients previously requiring frequent hospitalizations. The results found that the per-month costs for hospitalizations, emergency room visits, and home care fell from $2,836 per patient to $2,508 per patient, a savings of $328 per patient per month. (Source: Haggerty, M.C., Stockdale-Woolley, R., & Nair, S. (1991). Respi-Care: an innovative home care program for the patient with chronic osbstructive pulmonary disease. *Chest*, 100(3), 607-612.

Appendix B

**Occupational Therapy is Important
When You are in Need of Home Health Service**

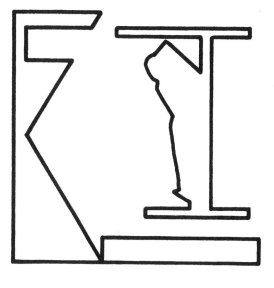

OCCUPATIONAL THERAPY is important when you are in need of

HOME HEALTH SERVICE

Facts for consumers from
*The American Occupational Therapy
Association, Inc.*

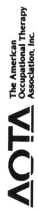

AOTA The American
Occupational Therapy
Association, Inc.

Finding home health services in your community

If you think you or a member of your family would benefit by receiving home health services, contact:

- your family physician
- hospitals in your community
- your local public health department
- your local home health agency.
- an occupational therapy practitioner, or

The American Occupational
Therapy Association, Inc.
4720 Montgomery Lane
PO Box 31220
Bethesda, MD 20824-1220

301-652-AOTA (2682)
301-652-7711 FAX
800-377-8555 TDD

It's not surprising to learn that people recovering from illness and injuries get better faster in their own homes. Everyday, more people are proving this thanks to the rapidly growing availability of home health services.

What are home health services?

These are specialized programs, which bring the services of professionals like occupational therapists, occupational therapy assistants, nurses, physical therapists, and speech and language pathologists to your home. Here, in familiar surroundings, you or your family member can continue your recovery and learn to deal with any remaining health or functional problems that could interfere with your ability to carry out daily tasks such as dressing, bathing, grooming, and cooking.

Who can benefit from home health services?

Home health services can be important in the treatment of people with limitations due to health or developmental problems such as those resulting from:

- Arthritis
- Heart disease
- Stroke
- Head injury
- Respiratory disease
- Hip fracture
- Cancer
- Parkinson's disease
- Diabetes
- Spinal cord injury
- Muscular dystrophy or multiple sclerosis
- Amyotrophic lateral sclerosis
- Developmental disability
- Cerebral palsy
- Burns

Occupational therapy can help at home by:

- working with you to aid you in being as independent as possible
- providing you with training and recommending equipment to help you care for your personal needs, such as bathing, dressing, and grooming
- identifying ways in which you can prepare and serve meals for yourself and your family
- teaching you how to make your home safer and more accessible when you must use a wheelchair, walker, or other aids and teaching you how to prevent injury or fatigue
- arranging supplies and equipment so you can continue your daily household tasks
- designing a program of activities and exercise that will help you regain as much function as possible
- working with you to decide upon the best ways to conserve energy and prevent injury and fatigue as you go about daily tasks
- constructing splints and adaptive equipment that will allow you to be as independent as possible
- aiding you in finding ways in which you can return to favorite leisure and recreational activities
- guiding you in planning for return to work and community life.

Who provides occupational therapy services?

Occupational therapy practitioners are trained health care professionals. The occupational therapist holds a bachelor's or master's degree and has completed a clinical internship. The occupational therapy assistant has an associate degree and has also completed a clinical internship. Both occupational therapists and occupational therapy assistants must pass a certification examination. Most states also regulate the practice of occupational therapy.

Payment for home health services

Home health services are covered under Medicare and are included as a covered service in many health insurance plans. Services may also be covered under insurance policies when you are injured in an auto accident or by workers' compensation if you are injured on the job. Contact your insurance company to determine coverage for your particular illness or disability.

Appendix C

Generic Home Health Agency Referral Form

Devised and developed by Karen Johnson, OTR

GENERIC HOME HEALTH AGENCY REFERRAL FORM

PATIENT NAME _____

ADDRESS_____ APT # _____

CITY/STATE/ZIP _____

PHONE_____ DOB _____ SEX_____

PRIMARY DIAGNOSIS_____ ONSET DATE _____

SECONDARY DIAGNOSIS/ONSET_____

SURGICAL PROCEDURES/DATES _____

MEDICATIONS _____

PHYSICIAN_____ PHONE _____

ADDRESS _____

PRIMARY CAREGIVER_____ RELATIONSHIP _____

HOME PHONE_____ WORK PHONE_____

CONTACT NAME_____ RELATIONSHIP _____

HOME PHONE_____ WORK PHONE_____

LAST HOSPITAL STAY FROM DATE_____ TO DATE _____

HOSPITAL NAME_____ HOSPITAL #_____

PAYOR SOURCE/# _____

REFERRAL SOURCE_____ TELEPHONE # _____

SN: ❏EVAL	AIDE:_____	❏MUSCLE RE-ED
❏VS, CV, CP, TEMP		❏ADAPT EQUIP
❏OBSV B/B STATUS	SW:_____	❏HOME ASSESS
❏NUTR/FL BAL		❏_____
❏MEDICATION	ST: ❏EVAL/TX	FREQ:_____
❏CK WEIGHT	❏LANG DIS TX	
❏CK BLOOD SUGAR	❏DYSPHAGIA TX	PT: ❏EVAL/TX
❏DRSNG CHNG	❏DYSPHASIA TX	❏ROM
❏PREFILL SYR	❏COGN RETRAIN	❏STRENGTHENING
❏PAIN CONTROL	❏_____	❏TRANSFERS
❏CK S/S INF/HEAL	FREQ:_____	❏GAIN TRAINING
❏CK NEURO STATUS		❏HEP
❏OSTOMY CARE	OT:❏EVAL/TX	❏ULTRASOUND
❏LAB WORK	❏ADL RETRAIN	❏SAFETY CHECK
❏CATH CARE	❏STRENGTHENING	❏HOME ASSESS
❏ADM IV/IM MEDS	❏ROM_____	❏_____
❏_____	❏FINE MOTOR	FREQ:_____
FREQ:_____	❏PERCEPT MOTOR	WBS_____

REMARKS/INSTRUCTIONS: _____

_____

_____

_____

_____

SIGNATURE_____ DATE _____

Appendix D

Coverage of Services

From the Department of Health and Human Services, Health Care Financing Administration, Medicare Home Health Agency Manual, Health Insurance Manual Publication 11, Section 205.2, Subsection D, April, 1989

205.2 <u>Skilled Therapy Services.</u>—

A. <u>General Principles Governing Reasonable and Necessary Physical Therapy, Speech Therapy, and Occupational Therapy.</u>—

1. The service of a physical, speech or occupational therapist is a skilled therapy service if the inherent complexity of the service is such that it can be performed safely and/or effectively only by or under the general supervision of a skilled therapist. To be covered, the skilled services must also be reasonable and necessary to the treatment of the beneficiary's illness or injury or to the restoration of maintenance of function affected by the beneficiary's illness or injury. It is necessary to determine whether individual therapy services are skilled and whether, in view of the beneficiary's overall condition, skilled management of the services provided is needed although many or all of the specific services needed to treat the illness or injury do not require the skills of a therapist.

2. The development, implementation management and evaluation of a patient care plan based on the physician's orders constitute skilled therapy services when, because of the beneficiary's condition, those activities require the involvement of a skilled therapist to meet the beneficiary's needs, promote recovery and ensure medical safety. Where the skills of a therapist are needed to manage and periodically reevaluate the appropriateness of a maintenance program because of an identified danger to the patient, such services would be covered, even if the skills of a therapist are not needed to carry out the activities performed as part of the maintenance program.

3. While a beneficiary's particular medical condition is a valid factor in deciding if skilled therapy services are needed, a beneficiary's diagnosis or prognosis should never be the sole factor in deciding that a service is or is not skilled. The key issue is whether the skills of a therapist are needed to treat the illness or injury, or whether the services can be carried out by nonskilled personnel.

4. A service that is ordinarily considered nonskilled could be considered a skilled therapy service in cases in which there is clear documentation that, because of special medical complications, skilled rehabilitation personnel are required to perform or supervise the service or to observe the beneficiary. However, the importance of a particular service to a beneficiary or the frequency with which it must be performed does not, by itself, make a nonskilled service into a skilled service.

5. The skilled therapy services must be reasonable and necessary to the treatment of the beneficiary's illness or injury within the context of the beneficiary's unique medical condition. To be considered reasonable and necessary for the treatment of the illness or injury:

a. The service must be consistent with the nature and severity of the illness or injury, the beneficiary's particular medical needs, including the requirement that the amount, frequency and duration of the services must be reasonable, and

b. The services must be considered, under accepted standards of medical practice, to be specific and effective treatment for the patient's condition, and

c. The services must be provided with the expectation, based on the assessment made by the physician of the beneficiary's rehabilitation potential, that:

+ The condition of the beneficiary will improve materially in a reasonable and generally predictable period of time, or

+ The services are necessary to the establishment of a safe and effective maintenance program.

Services involving activities for the general welfare of any beneficiary, e.g., general exercises to promote overall fitness or flexibility and activities to provide diversion or general motivation, do not constitute skilled therapy. Those services can be performed by nonskilled individuals without the supervision of a therapist.

d. Services of skilled therapists which are for the purpose of teaching the patient or the patient's family or caregivers necessary techniques, exercises or precautions are covered to the extent that they are reasonable and necessary to treat illness or injury. However, visits made by skilled therapists to a beneficiary's home solely to train other home health agency staff (e.g., home health aides) are not billable as visits since the home health agency is responsible for ensuring that its staff is properly trained to perform any service it furnishes. The cost of a skilled therapist's visit for the purpose of training home health agency staff is an administrative cost to the home health agency.

EXAMPLE: A beneficiary with a diagnosis of multiple sclerosis has recently been discharged from the hospital following an exacerbation of her condition which has left her wheelchair bound and, for the first time, without any expectation of achieving ambulation again. The physician has ordered physical therapy to select the proper wheelchair for her long term use, to teach safe use of the wheelchair and safe transfer techniques to the beneficiary and the family. Physical therapy would be reasonable and necessary to evaluate the beneficiary's overall needs, to make the selection of the proper wheelchair and to teach the beneficiary and/or family safe use of the wheelchair and proper transfer techniques.

   B. Application of the Principles to Physical Therapy Services.—The following discussion of skilled physical therapy services applies the principles in §205.2A to specific physical therapy services about which questions are most frequently raised.

      1. Assessment.—The skills of a physical therapist to assess a beneficiary's rehabilitation needs and potential or to develop and/or implement a physical therapy program are covered when they are reasonable and necessary because of the beneficiary's condition. Skilled rehabilitation services concurrent with the management of a patient's care plan include objective tests and measurements such as, but not limited to, range of motion, strength, balance coordination endurance or functional ability.

      2. Therapeutic Exercises.—Therapeutic exercises which must be performed by or under the supervision of the qualified physical therapist to ensure the safety of the beneficiary and the effectiveness of the treatment, due either to the type of exercise employed or to the condition of the beneficiary, constitute skilled physical therapy.

      3. Gait Training.—Gait evaluation and training furnished a beneficiary whose ability to walk has been impaired by neurological, muscular or skeletal abnormality require the skills of a qualified physical therapist and constitute skilled physical therapy and are considered reasonable and necessary if they can be expected to improve materially the beneficiary's ability to walk.

Gait evaluation and training which is furnished to a beneficiary whose ability to walk has been impaired by a condition other than a neurological, muscular or skeletal abnormality would nevertheless be covered where physical therapy is reasonable and necessary to restore the lost function.

EXAMPLE 1: A physician has ordered gait evaluation and training for a beneficiary whose gait has been materially impaired by scar tissue resulting from burns. Physical therapy services to evaluate the beneficiary's gait, to establish a gait training program and to provide the skilled services necessary to implement the program would be covered.

EXAMPLE 2: A beneficiary who has had a total hip replacement is ambulatory but demonstrates weakness, and is unable to climb stairs safely. Physical therapy would be reasonable and necessary to teach the beneficiary to safely climb and descend stairs.

Repetitive exercises to improve gait, or to maintain strength and endurance and assistive walking are appropriately provided by nonskilled persons and ordinarily do not require the skills of a physical therapist. Where such services are performed by a physical therapist as part of the initial design and establishment of a safe and effective maintenance program, the services would, to the extent that they are reasonable and necessary, be covered.

EXAMPLE: A beneficiary who has received gait training has reached his maximum restoration potential, and the physical therapist is teaching the beneficiary and family how to safely perform the activities which are a part of the maintenance program being established. The visits by the physical therapist to demonstrate and teach the activities (which by themselves do not require the skills of a therapist) would be covered since they are needed to establish the program.

      4. Range of Motion.—Only a qualified physical therapist may perform range of motion tests and therefore such tests are skilled physical therapy.

Range of motion exercises constitute skilled physical therapy only if they are part of an active treatment for a specific disease state, illness, or injury, which has resulted in a loss or restriction of mobility (as evidenced by physical therapy notes showing the degree of motion lost and the degree to be restored). Range of motion exercises which are not related to the restoration of a specific loss of function often may be provided safely and effectively by nonskilled individuals. Passive exercises to maintain range of motion in paralyzed extremities that can be carried out by nonskilled persons do not constitute skilled physical therapy.

However, as indicated in section 205.2A4, where there is clear documentation that, because of special medical complications (e.g., susceptible to pathological bone fractures), the skills of a therapist are needed to provide services which ordinarily do not need the skills of a therapist, then the services would be covered.

5. <u>Maintenance Therapy</u>.—Where repetitive services which are required to maintain function involve the use of complex and sophisticated procedures, the judgement and skill of a physical therapist might be required for the safe and effective rendition of such services. If the judgment and skill of a physical therapist is required to safely and effectively treat the illness or injury, the services would be covered as physical therapy services.

EXAMPLE: Where there is an unhealed, unstable fracture which requires regular exercise to maintain function until the fracture heals, the skills of a physical therapist would be needed to ensure that the fractured extremity is maintained in proper position and alignment during maintenance range of motion exercises.

Establishment of a maintenance program is a skilled physical therapy service where the specialized knowledge and judgement of a qualified physical therapist is required for the program to be safely carried out and the treatment aims of the physician achieved.

EXAMPLE: A Parkinson's patient or a patient with rheumatoid arthritis who has not been under a restorative physical therapy program may require the services of a physical therapist to determine what type of exercises are required for the maintenance of his present level of function. The initial evaluation of the patient's needs, the designing of a maintenance program which is appropriate to the capacity and tolerance of the patient and the treatment objectives of the physician, the instruction of the beneficiary, family or caregivers to safely and effectively carry out the program and such reevaluations as may be required by the beneficiary's condition, would constitute skilled physical therapy.

While a patient is under a restorative physical therapy program, the physical therapist should regularly reevaluate his condition and adjust any exercise program the patient is expected to carry out himself or with the aid of supportive personnel to maintain the function being restored. Consequently, by the time it is determined that no further restoration is possible (i.e., by the end of the last restorative session) the physical therapist will already have designed the maintenance program required and instructed the beneficiary or caregivers in carrying out the program.

6. <u>Ultrasound, Shortwave, and Microwave Diathermy Treatments</u>.—These treatments must always be performed by or under the supervision of a qualified physical therapist and are skilled therapy.

7. <u>Hot Packs, Infra-Red Treatments, Paraffin Baths and Whirlpool Baths</u>.—Heat treatments and baths of this type ordinarily do not require the skills of a qualified physical therapist. However, the skills, knowledge and judgment of a qualified physical therapist might be required in the giving of such treatments or baths in a particular case, e.g., where the patient's condition is complicated by circulatory deficiency, areas of desensitization, open wounds, fracture or other complications.

C. <u>Application of the General Principles to Speech Language Pathology Services</u>.—Speech pathology services are those services necessary for the diagnosis and treatment of speech and language disorders which result in communication disabilities and for the diagnosis and treatment of swallowing disorders (dysphagia), regardless of the presence of a communication disability. The following discussion of skilled speech language pathology services applies the principles to specific speech language pathology services about which questions are most frequently raised.

1. The skills of a speech language pathologist are required for the assessment of a beneficiary's rehabilitation needs (including the casual factors and the severity of the speech and language disorders), and rehabilitation potential. Reevaluation would only be considered reasonable and necessary if the beneficiary exhibited a change in functional speech or motivation, clearing of confusion or the remission of some other medical condition that previously contraindicated speech language pathology services. Where a beneficiary is undergoing restorative speech language pathology services, routine reevaluations are considered to be a part of the therapy and could not be billed as a separate visit.

2. The services of a speech language pathologist would be covered if they are needed as a result of an illness, or injury and are directed towards specific speech/voice production.

3. Speech language pathology would be covered where the service can only be provided by a speech language pathologist and where it is reasonably expected that the service will materially improve the beneficiary's ability to independently carry out any one or combination of communicative activities of daily living in a manner that is measurably at a higher level of attainment than that prior to the initiation of the services.

4. The services of a speech language pathologist to establish a hierarchy of speech-voice-language communication tasks and cuing that directs a beneficiary toward speech-language communication goals in the plan of care would be covered speech language pathology.

5. The services of a speech language pathologist to train the beneficiary, family or other caregivers to augment the speech-language communication, treatment or to establish an effective maintenance program would be covered speech therapy.

6. The services of a speech language pathologist to assist beneficiaries with aphasia in rehabilitation of speech and language skills is covered when needed by a beneficiary.

7. The services of a speech therapist to assist individuals with voice disorders to develop proper control of the vocal and respiratory systems for correct voice production are covered when needed by a beneficiary.

D. Application of the General Principles to Occupational Therapy.—The following discussion of skilled occupational therapy services applies the principles to specific occupational therapy services about which questions are most frequently raised.

1. Assessment.—The skills of an occupational therapist to assess and reassess a beneficiary's rehabilitation needs and potential or to develop and/or implement an occupational therapy program are covered when they are reasonable and necessary because of the beneficiary's condition.

2. Planning, Implementing and Supervision of Therapeutic Programs.—The planning, implementing and supervision of therapeutic programs including, but not limited to those listed below are skilled occupational therapy services, and if reasonable and necessary to the treatment of the beneficiary's illness or injury would be covered.

a. Selecting and teaching task oriented therapeutic activities designed to restore physical function.

EXAMPLE: Use of woodworking activities on an inclined table to restore shoulder, elbow and wrist range of motion lost as result of burns.

b. Planning, implementing and supervising therapeutic tasks and activities designed to restore sensory-integrative function.

EXAMPLE: Providing motor and tactile activities to increase sensory output and improve response for a stroke patient with functional loss resulting in a distorted boy image.

c. Planning, implementing and supervising of individualized therapeutic activity programs as part of an overall "active treatment" program for a patient with a diagnosed psychiatric illness.

EXAMPLE: Use of sewing activities which require following a pattern to reduce confusion and restore reality orientation in a schizophrenic patient.

d. Teaching compensatory techniques to improve the level of independence in the activities of daily living.

EXAMPLE: Teaching a beneficiary who has lost use of an arm how to pare potatoes and chop vegetables with one hand.

EXAMPLE: Teaching a stroke patient new techniques to enable him to perform feeding, dressing and other activities of daily living as independently as possible.

e. The designing, fabricating and fitting of orthotic and self-help devices.

EXAMPLE: Construction of a device which would enable an individual to hold a utensil and feed himself independently.

EXAMPLE: Construction of a hand splint for a patient with rheumatoid arthritis to maintain the hand in a functional position.

        f. Vocational and prevocational assessment and training which is directed toward the restoration of function in the activities of daily living lost due to illness or injury would be covered. Where vocational or prevocational assessment and training is related solely to specific employment opportunities, work skills or work settings, such services would not be covered because they would not be directed toward the treatment of an illness or injury.

        3. Illustration of Covered Services.—

EXAMPLE 1   :A physician orders occupational therapy for a patient who is recovering from a fractured hip and who needs to be taught compensatory and safety techniques with regard to lower extremity dressing, hygiene, toileting and bathing. The occupational therapist will establish goals for the beneficiary's rehabilitation (to be approved by the physician), and will undertake the teaching of the techniques necessary for the patient to reach the goals. Occupational therapy services would be covered at a duration and intensity appropriate to the severity of the impairment and the beneficiary's response to treatment.

EXAMPLE 2:   A physician has ordered occupational therapy for a beneficiary who is recovering from a CVA. The beneficiary has decreased range of motion, strength and sensation in both the upper and lower extremities on the right side. In addition, the beneficiary has perceptual and cognitive deficits resulting from the CVA. The beneficiary's condition has resulted in decreased function in activities of daily living (specifically bathing, dressing, grooming, hygiene and toileting). The loss of function requires assistive devices to enable the beneficiary to compensate for the loss of function and to maximize safety and independence. The beneficiary also needs equipment such as himi-slings to prevent shoulder subluxation and a hand splint to prevent joint contracture and deformity in the right hand.

        The services of an occupational therapist would be necessary to assess the beneficiary's needs, develop goals (to be approved by the physician), to manufacture or adapt the needed equipment to the beneficiary's use, to teach compensatory techniques, to strengthen the beneficiary as necessary to permit use of compensatory techniques, to provide activities which are directed towards meeting the goals governing increased perceptual and cognitive function. Occupational therapy services would be covered at ta duration and intensity appropriate to the severity of the impairment and the beneficiary's response to treatment.

206.   COVERAGE OF OTHER HOME HEALTH SERVICES

206.1 Skilled Nursing Care, Physical Therapy, Speech Therapy, and Occupational Therapy.—Where the beneficiary meets the qualifying criteria in 204, Medicare covers skilled nursing services which meet the requirements of 205.1 A and B and 206.7, physical therapy which meets the requirements of 205.2 A and B, speech therapy which meets the requirements of 205.2 A and C, and occupational therapy which meets the requirements of 205.2 A and D.

206.2 Home Health Aide Services.— For home health aide services to be covered, the beneficiary must meet the qualifying criteria as specified in §204, the services which are provided by the home health aide must be part-time or intermittent as discussed in §206.7; the services must meet the definition of home health aide services of this section; and the services must be reasonable and necessary to the treatment of the beneficiary's illness or injury.

The reason for the visits by the home health aide must be to provide hands-on personal care of the beneficiary or services which are needed to maintain the beneficiary's health or to facilitate treatment of the beneficiary's illness or injury.

The physician's order should indicate the frequency of the home health aide services required by the beneficiary. These services may include but are not limited to:

      a.   Personal Care.—Personal care means:

         •   Bathing, dressing, grooming, caring for hair, nail and oral hygiene which are needed to facilitate treatment or to prevent deterioration of the beneficiary's health, changing the bed linens of an incontinent beneficiary, shaving, deodorant application, skin care with lotions and/or powder, foot care, and ear care.

- Feeding, assistance with elimination (including enemas unless the skills of a licensed nurse are required due to the patient's condition, routine catheter care and routine colostomy care), assistance with ambulation, changing position in bed, assistance with transfers.

Appendix E

Occupational Therapy Assessment

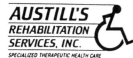

AUSTILL'S
REHABILITATION
SERVICES, INC.
SPECIALIZED THERAPEUTIC HEALTH CARE

OCCUPATIONAL THERAPY ASSESSMENT

Agency: _____ Date: _____

Patient Name:_____Therapist's Name: _____

Diagnosis/Background Information: _____

_____

_____

DOB: _____ Sex: ____ Precautions: _____

UPPER EXTREMITY PHYSICAL STATUS
WNL = within normal limits; **WFL** = within functional limits;
F = fair; **P** = poor **T** = trace; **0** = zero
Active ___ Passive ___

ROM JOINT	STRENGTH TONE (R)	STRENGTH TONE (L)	PAIN
SHOULDER			
ELBOW (Forearm)			
Wrist			
Thumb			

Comments: _____

SENSATION_____

_____

FINE MOTOR
Dominance ___ Grasp (R) ___ Grasp (L) ____
Finger Dexterity _____
Bilateral Coordination _____
Unilateral Coordination _____
Comments:_____

LOWER EXTREMITY FUNCTION

_____

_____

BALANCE
Sitting Unsupported _____
Sitting in W/C _____Standing _____
Ambulating _____
Comments: _____

ENDURANCE:_____

_____

_____

POSITIONING/EQUIPMENT: _____

_____

_____

I = Able to perform safely/independently/timely;
I/Device = modified independence (device); **S** = supervision;
Min. Assist (25%+ assist.); **Mod. Assist** (50%+ assist.); **Max.**
Assist (75%+ assist.); **D** = Dependent, Total Assist

POSITION CHANGES

Bed Mobility _____
Sit to Stand _____ W/C Manage. ____
Comments: _____

TRANSFERS

Bed _____ Toilet _____
Shower/Tub _____
Chair/Wheelchair _____
Comments: _____

COGNITIVE FUNCTION

Orientation _____
Attention Span _____
Understanding Directions _____
Communication _____
Memory _____
Problem Solving _____
Judgement/Safety _____
Motivation _____

Comments: _____

VISUAL/AUDITORY ABILITY

_____

_____

PERCEPTUAL PROCESSING

Body Scheme/Spatial Relations: _____

_____
Psychosocial Adjustment _____

LIVING ARRANGEMENTS

House ___ 1 story ___ 2 story Apartment ___
Bedroom Location _____ Hosp.Bed ___
Reg. Bed ___Steps/railings _____
Lives with _____
Safety _____
Cultural Environment: _____
Comments:_____

OCCUPATIONAL THERAPY ASSESSMENT

Patient Name: _____ Agency _____ Date _____

SELF CARE ABILITY
I = Able to perform safely/independently/timely;
I/Device = modified independence (device); **S** = supervision; **Min.
Assist.** (25%+ assist.); **Mod. Assist.**(50%+ assist.); **Max. Assist**
(75%+ assist.); **D** = Dependent, Total Assist

1. Oral Motor Control
_____
_____

2. Eating
Feeds Self _____
Drinks from Cup _____
Cuts with Knife_____
Opens Cartons_____
Brings food to table_____
Comments_____
_____

3. Dressing
Upper Body _____
Lower Body_____
Fasteners etc._____
Obtain Clothes-Closet/drawer_____
Comments_____
_____

4. Daily Routine_____
_____
_____

5. Bathing
Shower/Tub Bath_____
Sponge Bathing_____
Safety_____ _____
Assistant Devices _____
Comments _____

6. Grooming
Teeth Brushing
Care of Dentures _____
Hair Combing _____
Shaving_____
 Wash Face/Hands _____
Comments _____

7. Toileting
Continence _____Adjust Clothing
Clean Self _____Flush Toilet
Assistive Devices _____
Comments _____

8. Household Activities
Cook ____Simple Meal _____
Clean_____
Shopping _____
Comments _____

9. Transportation
Drive Self _____
Public Transportation _____
Comments _____

OVERALL SUMMARY

LONG TERM GOALS

SHORT TERM GOALS

TREATMENT PLAN (circle codes) D1-Eval.; D2-ADL; D3-Motor Re-ed.; D5-Percept Training; D6-Fine Coord.; D7- Neuro Training; D8-Sensory Training; D9-Orth/Splint; D10-Adapt.Equip.; D11-Other

FREQUENCY/DURATION

____ X WEEK ____ WEEKS

REHABILITATION POTENTIAL

DISCHARGE PLANS

Date:_____

Occupational Therapist:_____

Austill's Rehabilitation Services, Inc., 105 Coeway Lane, Exton, PA 19341-2203, (610) 363-7009

Appendix F

Individualized Education Program

Individualized Education Program

Name: John Doe   **School:** Oak Street

Grade: 1   **Exceptionality:** Learning Disabled

Present Level of Educational Performance:

1. John omits prepositional concepts when talking.
2. John confuses instructions that contain prepositional concepts, 100% of the time.
3. John draws shapes, but writes no letters.
4. John engages in sedentary play 100% of the time
5. John reads his first name and the word "go."

Special Education: Daily sessions in resource room for 1/2 hour.

Speech Therapy: Classroom contact with child and teacher twice a week for 20 minutes.

Occupational Therapy: Classroom contact with child and teacher for 1/2 hour once a week.

Regular Education: 88% of day—All classes except 1/2 hour resource daily.

Dates: 12/3/89 to 12/2/90.

Annual goals	Short-term instructional objectives
1. John will verbally use and comprehend five prepositions.	1. By January 15, 1990, John will spatially explore the classroom playscape by climbing over, under, onto, through, and around the playscape during free play observation by the classroom teacher ten days in a row.
	2. By February 28, 1990, John will correctly position himself in reference to classroom objects in response to verbal directions 100% of the time.
	3. By May 15, 1990, John will state where he is moving himself in reference to classroom objects with 100% accuracy using five different prepositions.

8-10

4. By December 2, 1990, John will place a pencil onto, beside, on top of, under, or through a cylinder in response to verbal commands with 100% accuracy.

2. John will read a six-word sentence.

1. By March 30, 1990, John will hold his head at midline and visually follow, with no loss of visual contact, a toy truck as it rolls across the table, as determined by skilled observation by the occupational therapist.

2. By September 30, 1990, John will read aloud six words with 100% accuracy three days in a row.

3. By December 2, 1990, John will read aloud the sentence, "I go to the big store," with 100% accuracy three days in a row.

3. John will write the alphabet.

1. By March 15, 1990, John will hold his pencil in a mature tripod pre-hension 100% of the time during ten randomly spaced observations by the teacher.

2. By May 15, 1990, when writing, John will sit on his desk chair with his feet on the floor and paper on the desk top, 100% of the time, during ten randomly spaced observations by the teacher.

3. By August 31, 1990, John will write, from example, one new letter a week using correct letter formation and spacing, with 100% accuracy.

4. By October 15, 1990, John will write, from dictation, four letters a week, using correct letter formation and spacing, with 100% accuracy.

5. By December 2, 1990, John will write the entire alphabet, from dictation, using a tripod grasp, while seated at his desk.

Appendix G

**Family Child Learning Center
Family Service Plan**

Family Child Learning Center
Family Service Plan

Plan # _____ of _____   Date: _____

Referral Date: _____ By Whom: _____ Coordinator: _____

Family Name: _____ Child's Name: _____

Address: _____ Phone: _____

Other Agencies Involved: _____

Family Members/Social Supports	Relationship

Child's Present Levels of Developmental Functioning: _____

Agency/Person	Contact Person	Phone

Outcomes:

#	Identified By?		Date:			

Family Needs/Resources Service/Action		Dates			
		Begin	Review	End	E

Infant Needs/Strengths Service/Action		Dates			
		Begin	Review	End	E

Outcomes:

#	Identified By?		Date:			

Family Needs/Resources Service/Action		Dates			
		Begin	Review	End	E

Infant Needs/Strengths Service/Action		Dates			
		Begin	Review	End	E

Appendix H

HCFA Form 485—

Home Health Certification and Plan of Care

HOME HEALTH CERTIFICATION AND PLAN OF CARE

1. Patient's HI Claim No.	2. Start Of Care Date	3. Certification Period		4. Medical Record No.	5. Provider No.
		From:	To:		

6. Patient's Name and Address

7. Provider's Name, Address and Telephone Number

8. Date of Birth	9. Sex ☐ M ☐ F	10. Medications: Dose/Frequency/Route (N)ew (C)hanged

11. ICD-9-CM	Principal Diagnosis	Date
12. ICD-9-CM	Surgical Procedure	Date
13. ICD-9-CM	Other Pertinent Diagnoses	Date

14. DME and Supplies	15. Safety Measures:
16. Nutritional Req.	17. Allergies:

18.A. Functional Limitations

1 ☐ Amputation	5 ☐ Paralysis	9 ☐ Legally Blind
2 ☐ Bowel/Bladder (Incontinence)	6 ☐ Endurance	A ☐ Dyspnea With Minimal Exertion
3 ☐ Contracture	7 ☐ Ambulation	B ☐ Other (Specify)
4 ☐ Hearing	8 ☐ Speech	

18.B. Activities Permitted

1 ☐ Complete Bedrest	6 ☐ Partial Weight Bearing	A ☐ Wheelchair
2 ☐ Bedrest BRP	7 ☐ Independent At Home	B ☐ Walker
3 ☐ Up As Tolerated	8 ☐ Crutches	C ☐ No Restrictions
4 ☐ Transfer Bed/Chair	9 ☐ Cane	D ☐ Other (Specify)
5 ☐ Exercises Prescribed		

19. Mental Status:

1 ☐ Oriented	3 ☐ Forgetful	5 ☐ Disoriented	7 ☐ Agitated
2 ☐ Comatose	4 ☐ Depressed	6 ☐ Lethargic	8 ☐ Other

20. Prognosis: 1 ☐ Poor 2 ☐ Guarded 3 ☐ Fair 4 ☐ Good 5 ☐ Excellent

21. Orders for Discipline and Treatments (Specify Amount/Frequency/Duration)

22. Goals/Rehabilitation Potential/Discharge Plans

23. Nurse's Signature and Date of Verbal SOC Where Applicable:	25. Date HHA Received Signed POT

24. Physician's Name and Address	26. I certify/recertify that this patient is confined to his/her home and needs intermittent skilled nursing care, physical therapy and/or speech therapy or continues to need occupational therapy. The patient is under my care, and I have authorized the services on this plan of care and will periodically review the plan.
27. Attending Physician's Signature and Date Signed	28. Anyone who misrepresents, falsifies, or conceals essential information required for payment of Federal funds may be subject to fine, imprisonment, or civil penalty under applicable Federal laws.

Form HCFA-485 (C-4) (02-94) (Print Aligned) **PROVIDER**

Privacy Act Statement

Sections 1812, 1814, 1815, 1816, 1861, and 1862 of the Social Security Act authorize collection of this information. The primary use of this information is to process and pay Medicare benefits to or on behalf of eligible individuals. Disclosure of this information may be made to : Peer Review Organizations and Quality Review Organizations in connection with their review of claims, or in connection with studies or other review activities, conducted pursuant to Part B of Title XI of the Social Security Act; State Licensing Boards for review of unethical practices or nonprofessional conduct; A congressional office from the record of an individual in response to an inquiry from the congressional office at the request of that individual.

Where the individual's identification number is his/her Social Security Number (SSN), collection of this information is authorized by Executive Order 9397. Furnishing the information on this form, including the SSN, is voluntary, but failure to do so may result in disapproval of the request for payment of Medicare benefits.

Paper Work Burden Statement

Public reporting burden for this collection of information is estimated to average 15 minutes per response and recordkeeping burden is estimated to average 15 minutes per response. This includes time for reviewing instructions, searching existing data sources, gathering and maintaining data needed, and completing and reviewing the collection of information. Send comments regarding this burden estimate or any other aspect of this collection of information, including suggestions for reducing the burden, to Health Care Financing Administration, P.O. Box 26684, Baltimore, Maryland 21207, and to the Office of Information and Regulatory Affairs, Office of Management and Budget, Washington, D.C. 20503. Paperwork Reduction Project 0938-0357.

Appendix H (cont'd.)

HCFA Form 486—
Home Health Certification and Plan of Care

Form Approved
OMB No. 0938-0357

MEDICAL UPDATE AND PATIENT INFORMATION

1. Patient's HI Claim No.	2. SOC Date	3. Certification Period		4. Medical Record No.	5. Provider No.
		From:	To:		

6. Patient's Name	7. Provider's Name

8. Medicare Covered: ☐ Y ☐ N	9. Date Physician Last Saw Patient:	10. Date Last Contacted Physician:

11. Is the Patient Receiving Care in an 1861 (J)(1) Skilled Nursing Facility or Equivalent?   ☐ Y ☐ N ☐ Do Not Know

12. ☐ Certification   ☐ Recertification   ☐ Modified

13. Specific Services and Treatments

Discipline	Visits (This Bill) Rel. to Prior Cert.	Frequency and Duration	Treatment Codes	Total Visits Projected This Cert.

14. Dates of Last Inpatient Stay: Admission Discharge	15. Type of Facility:

16. Updated Information: New Orders/Treatments/Clinical Facts/Summary from Each Discipline

17. Functional Limitations (Expand From 485 and Level of ADL) Reason Homebound/Prior Functional Status

18. Supplementary Plan of Treatment on File from Physician Other than Referring Physician:
(If Yes, Please Specify Giving Goals/Rehab. Potential/Discharge Plan)   ☐ Y ☐ N

19. Unusual Home/Social Environment

20. Indicate Any Time When the Home Health Agency Made a Visit and Patient was Not Home and Reason Why if Ascertainable	21. Specify Any Known Medical and/or Non-Medical Reasons the Patient Regularly Leaves Home and Frequency of Occurrence

22. Nurse or Therapist Completing or Reviewing Form	Date (Mo., Day, Yr.)

Form HCFA-486 (C3) (4-87)   **PROVIDER**

MEDICAL UPDATE AND PATIENT INFORMATION

1. Patient's HI Claim No.	2. SOC Date	3. Certification Period		4. Medical Record No.	5. Provider No.
		From:	To:		

6. Patient's Name	7. Provider's Name

8. Medicare Covered: ☐ Y ☐ N | 9. Date Physician Last Saw Patient: | 10. Date Last Contacted Physician:

11. Is the Patient Receiving Care in an 1861 (J)(1) Skilled Nursing Facility or Equivalent? ☐ Y ☐ N ☐ Do Not Know | 12. ☐ Certification ☐ Recertification ☐ Modified

13. Specific Services and Treatments

Discipline	Visits (This Bill) Rel. to Prior Cert.	Frequency and Duration	Treatment Codes	Total Visits Projected This Cert.

14. Dates of Last Inpatient Stay: Admission _____ Discharge _____ | 15. Type of Facility:

16. Updated Information: New Orders/Treatments/Clinical Facts/Summary from Each Discipline

17. Functional Limitations (Expand From 485 and Level of ADL) Reason Homebound/Prior Functional Status

18. Supplementary Plan of Treatment on File from Physician Other than Referring Physician: (If Yes, Please Specify Giving Goals/Rehab. Potential/Discharge Plan) ☐ Y ☐ N

19. Unusual Home/Social Environment

20. Indicate Any Time When the Home Health Agency Made a Visit and Patient was Not Home and Reason Why if Ascertainable	21. Specify Any Known Medical and/or Non-Medical Reasons the Patient Regularly Leaves Home and Frequency of Occurrence

22. Nurse or Therapist Completing or Reviewing Form	Date (Mo., Day, Yr.)

Form HCFA-486 (C3) (4-87)   **PHYSICIAN**

Appendix H (cont'd.)

HCFA Forms 485 and 486—accompanying documents

From Health Care Financing Administration, Department of Health and Human Services, Medicare Home Health Manual, Chapter II, page 24m4x7

EXHIBIT V

TREATMENT CODES FOR PROFESSIONAL SERVICES REQUIRED
Skilled Nursing

A1* Skilled Observation and Assessment
     (Inc. V.S., Response to Med., etc.)
A2 Foley Insertion
A3 Bladder Instillation
A4* Open Wound Care/Dressing
A5* Decubitus Care
     (Partial tissue loss with signs
     of infection or full thickness
     tissue loss etc.)
A6* Venipuncture
A7* Restorative Nursing
A8 Post Cataract Care
A9 Bowel/Bladder Training
A10 Chest Physio (Inc. Postural
     drainage)
A11 Adm. of Vitamin B/12
A12 Adm. Insulin
A13 Adm. Other IM/Subq.
A14 Adm. IV/s/Clysis

A15 Teach Ostomy or Ileo
     conduit care
A16 Teach Nasogastric Feeding
A17 Reinsertion Nasogastric
     Feeding Tube
A18 Teach Gastrostomy Feeding
A19 Teach Parenteral Nutrition
A20 Teach Care of Trach

A21 Adm. Care of Trach
A22* Teach Inhalation Rx
A23* Adm. Inhalation Rx
A24 Teach Adm. of Injection
A25 Teach Diabetic Care
A26 Disimpaction/F.U. Enema
A27* Other (Spec. under Orders)
A28* Wound Care/Dressing –
     Closed Incision/Suture Line
A29* Decubitus Care (Other than
     A5)
A30 Teaching Care of Any
     Indwelling Catheter
A31 Management and Evaluation
     of Patient Care Plan
A32* Teaching and Training
     (other) (spec. under order)

Physical Therapy

B1 Evaluation
B2 Therapeutic Exercise
B3 Transfer Training
B4 Home Program
B5

B6 Pulmonary Physical Therapy

B7 UltraSound
B8 Electrotherapy
B9 Prosthetic Training
B10 Fabrication   Temporary
    Gait Training Devices
B11 Muscle Re-education
B12 Management and Evaluation
    of a Patient Care Plan
B13-14 Reserved
B15* Other (Specify   under

orders)

Speech Therapy

C1 Evaluation
C2 Voice Disorders Treatments
C3 Speech Articulation Disorders
     Treatments
C4 Dysphagia Treatments
C5 Language Disorders Treatments

C6 Aural Rehabilitation
C7 Reserved
C8 Nonoral Communication
C9* Other (Specify under
     Orders)

*Code which requires a more extensive descriptive narrative for physician's
orders.

Exhibit V (Cont.)   MEDICAL REVIEW   09-94

Occupational Therapy

D1   Evaluation
D2   Independent Living/Daily Living Skills (ADL Training)
D3   Muscle Re-education
D4   Reserved
D5   Perceptual Motor Training
D6   Fine Motor Coordination
D7   Neuro-developmental Treatment
D8   Sensory Treatment
D9   Orthotics/Splinting
D10 Adaptive Equipment (fabrication and training)
D11* Other (Specify Under Orders)

Medical Social Services

E1   Assessment of Social and Emotional Factors
E2   Counseling for Long Range Planning and Decision Making
E3   Community Resource Planning
E4* Short Term Therapy
E5   Reserved
E6* Other (Specify Under Orders)

Home Health Aide

F1	Tub/Shower Bath	F8	Assist with Ambulation
F2	Partial/Complete Bed Bath	F9	Reserved
F3	Reserved	F10	Exercises
F4	Personal Care	F11	Prepare Meal
F5	Reserved	F12	Grocery Shop
F6	Catheter Care	F13	Wash Clothes
F7	Reserved	F14	Housekeeping
		F15*	Other (Spec. under Orders)

*Code which requires a more extensive descriptive narrative for physician's orders.

Appendix H (cont'd.)

HCFA Forms 485 and 486—accompanying documents

From Health Care Financing Administration, Department of Health and Human Services, Medicare Home Health Manual, Section 234.9, pages 24m4o–24m4p

o **C3.   Speech Articulation Disorders Treatments** - Procedures and treatment for patients with impaired intelligibility (clarity) of speech - usually referred to as anarthria or dysarthria and/or impaired ability to initiate, inhibit, and/or sequence speech sound muscle movements - usually referred to as apraxia/dyspraxia.

o **C4.   Dysphagia Treatments** - Includes procedures designed to facilitate and restore a functional swallow.

o **C5.   Language Disorders Treatments** - Includes procedures and treatment for patients with receptive and/or expressive aphasia/dysphasia, impaired reading comprehension, written language expression, and/or arithmetical processes.

o **C6. Aural Rehabilitation** - Procedures and treatments designed for patients with communication problems related to impaired hearing acuity.

o **C7.   Reserved**

o **C8.   Nonoral Communications** - Includes any procedures designed to establish a non-oral or augmentive communication system.

o **C9. Other (Spec. Under Orders)** - Speech therapy services not included above. Specify service to be rendered under physician's orders (HCFA-485 Item 21).

D. **Occupational Therapy.**--These codes represent the services to be rendered by the occupational therapist. Following is a further explanation:

o **D1. Evaluation** - Visit made to determine occupational therapy needs of the patient at the home. Includes physical and psychosocial testings, establishment of plan of care, rehabilitation goals, and evaluating the home environment for accessibility and safety and recommending modifications.

o **D2.   Independent Living/Daily Living Skills (ADL training)** - Refers to the skills and performance of physical cognitive and psychological/emotional self care, work, and play/leisure activities to a level of independence appropriate to age, life-space, and disability.

o **D3. Muscle Re-education** - Includes therapy designed to restore function lost due to disease or surgical intervention.

o **D4.   Reserved**

o **D5.   Perceptual Motor Training** - Refers to enhancing skills necessary to interpret sensory information so that the individual can interact normally with the environment. Training designed to enhance perceptual motor function usually involves activities which stimulate visual and kinesthetic channels to increase awareness of the body and its movement.

o **D6.   Fine Motor Coordination** - Refers to the skills and the performance in fine motor and dexterity activities.

o **D7. Neurodevelopmental Treatment** - Refers to enhancing the skills and the performance of movement through eliciting and/or inhibiting stereotyped, patterned, and/or involuntary responses which are coordinated at subcortical and cortical levels.

o **D8. Sensory Treatment** - Refers to enhancing the skills and performance in perceiving and differentiating external and internal stimuli such as tactile awareness, stereognosis, kinesthesia, proprioceptive awareness, ocular control, vestibular awareness, auditory awareness, gustatory awareness, and factory awareness necessary to increase function.

o **D9. Orthotics/Splinting** - Refers to the provision of dynamic and static splints, braces, and slings for relieving pain, maintaining joint alignment, protecting joint integrity, improving function, and/or decreasing deformity.

o **D10. Adaptive Equipment (fabrication and training)** - Refers to the provision of special devices that increase independent functions.

o **D11. Other** - Occupational therapy services not quantified above.

E. **Medical Social Services (MSS)**.--These codes represent the services to be rendered by the medical social service worker. Following is a further explanation:

o **E1. Assessment of Social and Emotional Factors** - Skilled assessment of social and emotional factors related to the patient's illness, need for care, response to treatment and adjustment to care; followed by care plan development.

o **E2. Counseling for Long-Range Planning and Decisionmaking** - Assessment of patient's needs for long term care including: evaluation of home and family situation; enabling patient/family to develop an inhome care system; exploring alternatives to inhome care; arrangement for placement.

o **E3. Community Resource Planning** - The promotion of community centered services(s) including education, advocacy, referral and linkage.

o **E4. Short Term Therapy** - Goal oriented intervention directed toward management of terminal illness; reaction/adjustment to illness; strengthening family/support system; conflict resolution related to chronicity of illness.

o **E5. Reserved**

o **E6. Other (Specify Under Orders)** - Includes other medical social services related to the patient's illness and need for care. Problem resolution associated with high risk indicators endangering patient's mental and physical health including: abuse/neglect; inadequate food/medical supplies; high suicide potential. The service to be performed must be written under doctor's orders, (HCFA-485, Item 21).

24m4p

Resources

Home Health Organizations

American Association for Continuity of Care
11250 Roger Bacon Drive
Suite 8
Reston, VA 22090-5202
(703) 437-4377

American Federation of Home Health Agencies
1320 Fenwick Lane
Suite 100
Silver Spring, MD 20910
(301) 588-1454

American Hospital Association
840 North Lake Shore Drive
Chicago, IL 60611
(312) 280-6708

American Medical Association
515 North State Street
Chicago, Il 60610
(312) 464-4755

The American Occupational Therapy Association
4720 Montgomery Lane
P.O. Box 31220
Bethesda, MD 20824-1220
(301) 652-2682

American Public Health Association
1015 15th Street, NW
Washington, DC 20005
(202) 789-5672

National Association for Home Care
519 C Street, NE
Stanton Park
Washington, DC 20002
(202) 547-7474

Health Industry Distributors Association
225 Reinekers Lane
Suite 650
Alexandria, VA 22314-2875
(703) 549-4432

Home Health Services and Staffing Association
115-D South St. Asaph Street
Alexandria, VA 22314
(703) 836-9863

National Association of Medical Equipment Suppliers
625 Slaters Lane
Suite 200
Alexandria, VA 22314-1171
(703) 836-6263

National League for Nursing
350 Hudson Street
4th Floor
New York, NY 10019
(212) 989-9393

Visiting Nurse Associations of America
3801 East Florida Avenue
Suite 900
Denver, CO 80210
(303) 753-0218

Home Health Publications

Home Health Line
1300 Rockville Pike
#1100
Rockville, MD 20852-3030
(301) 816-8950

Hospital Home Health
American Health Consultants, Inc.
67 Peachtree Park Drive, NE
Atlanta, GA 30309
(404) 351-4523

Independent Living Provider
Equal Opportunity Publications
150 Motor Parkway
Happauge, NY 11788
(516) 273-0066

Journal of Home Health Practice
Aspen Publications
7201 McKinney Circle
Frederick, MD 21701
(800) 234-1660

National Association of Medical Equipment Suppliers
625 Slaters Lane
Suite 200
Alexandria, VA 22314-1171
(703) 836-6263

National League for Nursing
350 Hudson Street
4th Floor
New York, NY 10019
(212) 989-9393

Visiting Nurse Associations of America
3801 East Florida Avenue
Suite 900
Denver, CO 80210
(303) 753-0218

Home Health Publications

Home Health Line
1300 Rockville Pike
#1100
Rockville, MD 20852-3030
(301) 816-8950

Hospital Home Health
American Health Consultants, Inc.
67 Peachtree Park Drive, NE
Atlanta, GA 30309
(404) 351-4523

Independent Living Provider
Equal Opportunity Publications
150 Motor Parkway
Happauge, NY 11788
(516) 273-0066

Journal of Home Health Practice
Aspen Publications
7201 McKinney Circle
Frederick, MD 21701
(800) 234-1660

Resources

Home Health Organizations

American Association for Continuity of Care
11250 Roger Bacon Drive
Suite 8
Reston, VA 22090-5202
(703) 437-4377

American Federation of Home Health Agencies
1320 Fenwick Lane
Suite 100
Silver Spring, MD 20910
(301) 588-1454

American Hospital Association
840 North Lake Shore Drive
Chicago, IL 60611
(312) 280-6708

American Medical Association
515 North State Street
Chicago, Il 60610
(312) 464-4755

The American Occupational Therapy Association
4720 Montgomery Lane
P.O. Box 31220
Bethesda, MD 20824-1220
(301) 652-2682

American Public Health Association
1015 15th Street, NW
Washington, DC 20005
(202) 789-5672

National Association for Home Care
519 C Street, NE
Stanton Park
Washington, DC 20002
(202) 547-7474

Health Industry Distributors Association
225 Reinekers Lane
Suite 650
Alexandria, VA 22314-2875
(703) 549-4432

Home Health Services and Staffing Association
115-D South St. Asaph Street
Alexandria, VA 22314
(703) 836-9863